Old Age in a New Age

The Promise

of Transformative Nursing Homes

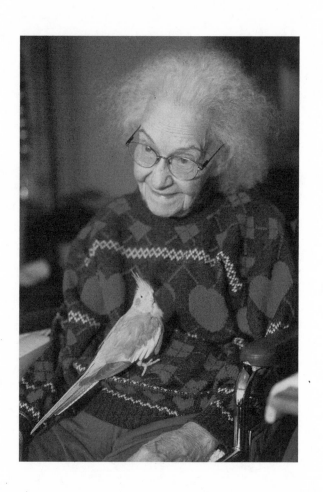

Old Age in a New Age

The Promise of Transformative Nursing Homes

Beth Baker

Vanderbilt University Press
Nashville

11 10 09 08   3 4 5

Printed on acid-free paper.
Manufactured in the United States of America
Designed by Dariel Mayer

Frontispiece: The late Lois Marie Newman at Bigfork Valley
Communities in 2003. Photo by Ross Wells.

Library of Congress Cataloging-in-Publication Data

Old age in a new age : the promise of transformative nursing homes /
Beth Baker.—1st ed.
p. ; cm.
Includes bibliographical references and index.
ISBN 13: 978-0-8265-1562-9 (cloth : alk. paper)
ISBN 13: 978-0-8265-1563-6 (pbk. : alk. paper)
1. Nursing homes—United States. 2. Older people—Nursing home
care—United States. 3. Older people—United States—Social condi-
tions—21st century. I. Title.
[DNLM: 1. Homes for the Aged—organization & administration—
United States. 2. Nursing Homes—organization & administration—
United States. 3. Aged—psychology—United States. 4. Organizational
Case Studies—United States. 5. Quality of Life—United States. WT 27
AA1 B1670 2007]
RA997.B323 2007
362.160973—dc22
2006038878

To our elders and those
who lovingly care for them

Contents

Acknowledgments

F irst, I wish to thank the elders, their families, staff, and administrators of
    nursing homes who welcomed me and shared their stories. Their kind-
ness, honesty, and good humor inspired this book. Charlene Boyd, Heidi Gil,
Steve Shields, and Bill Thomas were particularly generous with their time
and supportive of my efforts. I am grateful to the leaders of the Pioneer
Network, Action Pact, Inc., and the National Citizens' Coalition for Nursing
Home Reform who shared their history and insights with me over the four
years I worked on the book. Their help was invaluable, as was that of the
many academic researchers whose knowledge is reflected here. If there are
any errors in these pages, they are my own.

My editors at the *Washington Post* Health section gave me assignments
that started me on this journey.

I am grateful to dear friends and family members, too numerous to name
here, who believed in this project and boosted my spirits. To my mother,
Betty, who, along with my late father, Bob, taught me to love the written
word, a special thanks. My sister, Bobbie, shared contacts in the Ohio Psychological Association, but more important gave me her unwavering confidence.
My sister-in-law, Dena Crosson, helped me gather important research materials. Friends who assisted me during the writing process included Barbara
Armstrong, Michael Culliton, Frank Gallant, Karen Gallant, Leah Glasheen,
Naomi Lubick, Bruce Johansen, Katie Pugliese, and Lynne Waymon. Anne
and Jim Williams twice generously loaned me their home on Long Cove so
that I might write without interruption. My daughter, Sarah, made helpful
suggestions as I developed the proposal, and she and my son, Danny, cheered
me on. The expert editorial eyes and enthusiasm of both Sara Taber and Sam
Horn were especially encouraging.

I also want to acknowledge Lillian Morrison for giving me permission
to reprint her poem, "Nursing Home," that first appeared in her wonderful
collection *A Good Catch for the Universe* (2005).

Thanks to my agent, Jodie Rhodes, and to Michael Ames at Vanderbilt University Press, who both embraced my book with enthusiasm from the moment they saw the proposal. Michael's support remained strong throughout the process, for which I am very grateful.

Finally, my deepest gratitude to my husband, Ross—my best friend, benefactor, and biggest booster—for his steadfast belief in my work.

Prologue

My grandma Sara always worked "in chocolate," as she put it, either making chocolates for Maud Muller Candies or selling chocolates at Rikes Department Store in Dayton, Ohio. She worked until she was in her eighties. Every birthday, I got my own two-pound box of Maud Mullers, filled with creams, toffees, and caramels, each nestled in a brown fluted-paper cup. My favorite gift is still a box of chocolates.

We kids adored Grandma. She seemed to get a kick out of life, accepting the hand that she was dealt. She had lost my grandfather, the love of her life, to lung cancer when he was in his fifties. But I never heard a word of self-pity from her.

She had little money, but she knew how to have fun. Weighing in at ninety pounds, she was stylish, wearing sling-back high heels, fashionable dresses, and gold costume jewelry, including a charm bracelet with a silhouette of each grandchild dangling from it. When she told a funny story, her laughter was punctuated with a snort. She grew flourishing roses and collected Hummel figurines.

I loved exploring the depths of her basement, which held an amazing octagonal table for playing cards, and the dark corners of her attic. My sister, brother, and I slept up there, in a brass bed on a lumpy mattress.

Grandma played endless games of canasta and euchre with us. She let me fix her hair in pin curls and administer facials, slathering her lined skin with concoctions of perfumed creams I mixed from bottles on her dresser. Never mind that she had just come from the beauty parlor—she always indulged us, just as her own parents had done with her, and as my father continued with us.

When Grandma was ninety-two, she decided she was too frail to live on her own. She had already given up the house on Kipling Drive and moved to an apartment. But when that became too much for her, she entered a nursing home. Once Grandma crossed the threshold, she seemed to fade away and be replaced by a generic old person. I knew she was happy to see us, but the spark was gone. I wondered if the staff even knew that she had worked in chocolate and could play countless varieties of poker.

The last time I saw her was shortly before she died in 1982. I was then thirty and indulging my own Sarah. My husband, Ross, and I took our two-year-old to see her namesake in the nursing home.

It was like most such institutions back then—and now, in far too many cases. To enter, we passed through a glass door and were met with the malodor of medicine, Mr. Clean, and urine. A long hall of linoleum led to the hospital-like rooms where residents lived.

Our daughter was knee-high, with wispy blond hair and sturdy legs. In a photo taken that day, she wears a dark blue jumper with embroidered flowers. A serious child, she was not the kind to make a ruckus. She held my hand as we made our way through the lobby. To do so, we passed a phalanx of very old women wearing faded housedresses or hospital gowns, sitting in wheelchairs. In my mind's eye, they moved as one long pale organism, leaning out of their chairs, quavering arms outstretched, painful yearning on their faces, to touch our daughter. I could feel their hunger for life, as represented by a small child.

If she was frightened by this display, Sarah did not show it. She solemnly submitted to the touch of these strangers as if she knew she was giving them a gift.

The haunting vision of elderly women grasping at life beyond their reach was frozen in my mind for the next twenty years. I never considered there could be an alternative for those who live in a nursing home. But wiser people, with far more imagination, are challenging the way we've done things. They are creating homes where people with physical or mental frailties live not as wards, patients, or inmates, but as contributing, creative human beings. These visionary leaders demonstrate that radically changing the culture of nursing homes transforms the lives of both elders and caregivers.

"The people in long-term care are the elders of our people," said Barry Barkan, a California leader in this emerging movement for social change. "They're growing, learning, developing. We believe that they still have potential, and that they deserve respect and honor. They still have a birthright to happiness, joy, and pleasure. And they have work to do, which is to formulate a legacy."

Would the end of my grandmother's life have been different had she lived in a home with such a philosophy? It's hard to know. But perhaps she would have kept her spark, dealing cards with new friends and laughing until the end.

Introduction

> The shift from the old culture to the new is not a matter of
> adding on a few items that were missing, but of seeing almost
> every feature in a different way.
> —Tom Kitwood, *Dementia Reconsidered*

I came to this story in a roundabout way, while writing a piece for the *Washington Post* on an unusual line of medical research. Scientists were quantifying what many people feel instinctively—that there are health benefits to being around nature. As part of my reporting, I tracked down Dr. Bill Thomas. He and his wife, Jude, had created a new kind of nursing home, one enriched with houseplants, a vegetable garden, cats, dogs, birds, and children. He called this model the Eden Alternative. By the time I interviewed him in 2002, he had won many converts to the radical notion that people in nursing homes could lead rich, rewarding lives.

Here was a much larger story than my original one. As Bill Thomas put it, "How do you take something as sterile, as institutional, as a nursing home and inject this normal pulse of life into it? That is the challenge."

Our conversation stayed with me. I went on to write articles about the movement, of which Bill Thomas is a part, to transform how we live in old age. The more I learned, the more I wanted to know. The leaders of this movement intrigued me. Bill Thomas, a blue-jeaned Harvard-educated physician, lives off the grid in rural New York and calls himself a nursing home "abolitionist." Steve Shields, a former oil prospector turned nursing home administrator, is the all-American can-do guy who led a nationally recognized transformation of a retirement community in Kansas. Charlene Boyd, sophisticated and dynamic, helped create a vibrant community of staff and elders at a Catholic long-term care facility in Seattle, and Eric Haider, an earnest, India-born visionary, turned a county poor farm in rural Missouri into one of the most liberated nursing homes in the country.

Their backgrounds, stories, and organizations were unique. Yet somehow, independent of each other, they arrived at similar strategies for transforming the lives of both residents and staff of nursing homes. They hope to be in the vanguard of a fundamental cultural shift in our society.

Eldercare in our country is a patchwork of housing and health services that includes short-term rehabilitation facilities, intermediate and skilled care, assisted living, small board-and-care homes, home-health services, adult daycare, and continuing-care retirement communities offering a spectrum of options. In this book, I focus on two important pieces of this patchwork—nursing homes and, to a lesser extent, assisted living. In part, this is where the trail of the story led me. But I also recognized that nursing homes are the most intractable and dreaded of these places. If we can find a way to make them right, the rest will fall into place.

I make an underlying assumption: that we will continue to need places where elders live, beyond their own homes. This may not be a bad thing. For many people living in their own home means being isolated, lonely, and fearful, eating microwaved frozen dinners and watching endless hours of television. Is it possible that one reason people cling to their independence is that the alternatives are so unappealing? What if instead there were communities where the spirit was nourished, along with the body tended?

Many assume that any significant change in eldercare is unaffordable. But as we will see, living well doesn't have to cost more. The places I visited served all classes of people, from those who were formerly homeless to those who were wealthy. Most places had a high proportion of residents who were on Medicaid.

Fundamentally, the envisioned change is one of the heart, and the investment that is required is not so much financial as attitudinal. Culture-change leaders address critical and costly problems such as high staff turnover and resident neglect. Exceptional homes also tend to have long waiting lists rather than empty rooms. By reducing expenses and increasing revenue, these homes do not typically cost more to operate.

That said, a foundational goal of any long-term care system should be a living wage and health insurance for all employees. Those who care for our most vulnerable loved ones deserve at least this much.

We—as taxpayers and as families—already pay an incredibly high price for places that we fear. Shouldn't we be getting something better for our money?

In writing the book, I drew on voluminous research on long-term care and aging. But I am not a social scientist, and this is not an academic text. Nor is it a manual, or a field guide to nursing homes. Readers will not find any rankings here, but rather a philosophy and approach. If you are search-ing for good options for a loved one, this book will prompt questions as you visit nursing homes or assisted-living centers. Indeed, by demanding better alternatives, we will help accelerate the movement for change.

I visited more than two dozen homes around the country and conducted phone interviews at many more. Many of them are part of the Pioneer Net-work, a coalition dedicated to changing the culture of aging and of nurs-ing homes. Others, most notably Kendal, a Quaker chain, were founded on a philosophy of honoring the dignity of every person and do not consider themselves part of any movement. Rose Marie Fagan, director of the Pioneer Network, and consultant LaVrene Norton of Action Pact guided me to homes they considered on the cutting edge of change. Others I discovered on my own. I sought a representative mix of places geographically that spanned the spectrum, from serving primarily low-income people on Medicaid through those that served wealthier, private-pay clients. While most are nonprofit, I also found for-profit homes striving to make deep change. Many wonderful places are not mentioned here, and at least one I visited has since backslid. Thus anyone considering one of the homes I describe should visit and ask questions of their own.

The vast majority of nursing home residents are elderly, and my book is directed at improving the lives of elders. I apologize to younger residents of nursing homes, who may not see their lives reflected in these pages. In truth, though, the small number of residents who are younger benefit equally from the changes under way.

I use individuals' real names, except when a name is enclosed in quota-tion marks. Unless otherwise cited, all quotes came from my interviews. I am deeply grateful for the openness of those I interviewed.

Every home I visited would describe itself as a work-in-progress or as on a journey. Yet some are much farther on the road. I draw on examples of those just beginning the process of change and those that were pioneers a decade ago. Some homes were stronger in one area than another: breaking the barriers between the outside world and the nursing home, for example, or renovating old hospital wings into genuine households. And while none claims to be perfect, to me the ones that had arrived at a meaningful way sta-tion on the journey were those that made me feel happy when I entered. Just that—I felt happy to be there. That quality cannot be measured or regulated. But it is powerful nonetheless.

I have come to believe that we have exhausted the regulatory answers to the conundrum of eldercare. While we should continue to push for com-pliance with high standards, the path to deep systemic change does not lie through the thicket of regulations, but rather in a new vision that is hopeful and realistic. As Benyamin Schwarz noted in his book on nursing home design: "What was reasonable to one era becomes almost incomprehensible to other eras. Despite its short life, it seems that the nursing home as an entity for the provision of long-term care for the elderly is a model from a different era that outlived its time."[1]

Nursing home administrator Steve Shields calls the warehousing of older people in nursing homes "the sin of the twentieth century," a sin for which we are all responsible. To continue with the religious metaphor, I believe he and others offer a path for redemption. It requires uprooting the institutional nature of the nursing home and planting in its place a new community that looks and feels much more like a home than a hospital, both in its physical design and in the relationships it nurtures. Today in our nation, hundreds of homes seek to do just that.

The stories in this book point us toward new ways of thinking and of being in relationship. Little miracles are taking place every day. People who have given up on themselves—or felt others had given up them—reawaken to life. Workers who were resentful and disrespected feel enthusiastic and creative about their jobs. Adult children once plagued with guilt for abandoning their parents feel grateful for the kindness and dignity their loved ones enjoy. I have been privileged to hear stories from people who are moved to tears about their work, and I have witnessed countless examples of older people's lives filled with humor, growth, and affection.

The challenge is whether these amazing places will remain rare jewels or become the norm. There is no reason they cannot be made available to all who need them. But that will not happen by itself. The lumbering system of regulation and reimbursement and the societal bias against aging will not be easy to turn around. It will take clear commitment and intentionality to replace our mass denial. Perhaps baby boomers will act in all our interests to force deep change.

We all have a stake in the lives of elders, whether they are beloved family members, neighbors, members of our church, or—us. Most of us will grow old, and many of us will need some sort of assistance. What would we want for ourselves? What is our vision of a good old age?

PART I

The Last Resort

The Glentyre Nursing Home was much as
these places are. . . . The same satellite TV
goes unwatched: chairs, though they may
begin informally grouped, end up with their
backs to the wall, where the occupants insist
that they be. Even a slight touch of paranoia
is enough to make you want to keep an eye on
what the others in the room are doing. Safer
not to have your back to anyone. The same
smell seeped into the very fabric of the walls,
of urine and disinfectant and old-fashioned
face powder. The same staff: a few cheerful
and kind, most sullen and underpaid. The
same sense of waiting, of bemusement that
life has come to this. Communal (that is to say,
lowest common denominator) taste when it
comes to the colour of walls and drapes. The
food provides nothing that anyone is likely to
object to, a consideration which more than
anything leaves the flavour of sadness in the
mouth. What we value all our life, what fires
us and sparks us, the sense of our individuality,
dampened down, crushed, deprived of oxygen.
No outrage allowed.
                    —Fay Weldon, *Rhode Island Blues*

Chapter 1

"Promise You'll Never Put Me in a Nursing Home"
Why We're in Denial

In ten years of research, no data has emerged to counteract my impression of nursing homes as death sentences, the final interment from which there is no exit but death.
> —Betty Friedan, *The Fountain of Age*

The time has arrived to let [the nursing home] go. It's time to let it go. Some would say it's broken. I say it never was fixed. It was never a healthy nourishing thing.
> —Steve Shields, nursing home administrator

For decades, aging parents have begged their children, "Promise you'll never put me in a nursing home." Older people declare they will never move to one—as if by stating it emphatically enough, they can protect themselves from this terrible fate. Indeed, many seriously ill older people say they would rather be dead than live in a nursing home—that is, until the time comes.[1]

Oddly, for more than half a century, we have lived with this state of affairs. We act as if the nursing home were an immutable part of life, like drought or disease, something to be regretted but accepted. Most of us haven't considered there might be a better way for frail, old, or disabled people to spend the rest of their lives. There, we think, but for the grace of God . . .

The nursing home as we know it is entrenched in our imaginations, our landscape, and our economy. There are thousands more nursing homes than McDonald's restaurants in the United States—17,000 compared to 12,468 Golden Arches in 2006.[2] Chances are you routinely drive by a nursing home and don't even notice it. They are often nondescript brick buildings with tidy grounds and no signs of life. Their names tend to reflect a nature theme—Autumnwoods, Springview, Magnolia Glen. But little is natural about life in a traditional nursing home.

In these facilities live 1.6 million people, with another 900,000 in assisted living, cared for by 2.7 million employees—twice the number employed at Wal-Marts in our country. Nursing homes alone cost the nation $111 billion annually. And the baby boomers haven't hit old age. The U.S. Census Bureau projects that the number of older people will double between 2000 and 2030, from 35 million to 72 million. By 2030, at current levels of use, 3 million people will live in nursing homes, according to the National Center for Health Statistics (NCHS).[3] Already 4.5 million people have Alzheimer's disease; by 2025 that number is expected to double, and it may double again by 2050, according to the Alzheimer's Association. Unless in the very near future medical researchers find ways to delay or treat major age-related illnesses, we can expect a sharp rise in the need for eldercare.

Who lives in assisted living and in nursing homes? For the most part, very frail old women who have no relatives able to assist them full-time. Ten percent are African American and 89 percent white; nearly 3 percent speak a language other than English. According to NCHS, growing numbers of people in nursing homes reflect the diverse ethnicity of our nation, a trend that is expected to continue. A small percentage of those in nursing homes are younger people with severe disabilities.

In general, nursing home residents are older and sicker than were nursing home residents in the past. On average, they are eighty-five or older, with three or more admitting diagnoses, the most common being cardiovascular disease and dementia. Other mental disorders, such as depression and anxiety, are common. People in nursing homes require some level of medical care, such as medication management or physical therapy, and many need help with everyday activities, such as bathing or eating. Most use wheelchairs. In addition to the long-term population, a growing number of people recovering from surgery, falls, or acute illness also spend some time in a nursing home.

Many people who once would have lived in a nursing home now live in assisted living. Billed as the anti-nursing home, assisted living promises older people a more independent and homey environment than a nursing facility offers. Assisted-living residents have their own small apartments but can get daily assistance with activities such as dressing or bathing. Most assisted-living residents pay out of pocket for this freedom, compared to the majority of nursing home residents whose care is covered through Medicaid.

Caring for old people is big business. In 2006, the average annual cost for private pay residents in a nursing home was nearly $71,000 for a private room, and $62,500 for a semiprivate room; a one-bedroom assisted-living unit cost more than $32,000 a year, not counting one-time entry fees. Two-thirds of nursing homes are for-profit enterprises, most of them operated by large corporations such as Kindred Healthcare and HCR/ManorCare. Of the not-for-profit nursing homes, most are church affiliated and a small number are government run. Nursing homes typically depend on a mix of private pay and Medicaid reimbursement, with private rates higher than what Medicaid pays. Nearly 15 percent of nursing homes, though, depend almost entirely on Medicaid for reimbursement, according to Brown University researcher Vincent Mor and his colleagues.[4] These homes, found in poor communities around the nation, are unable to attract and keep competent staff in adequate numbers, no matter how good their intentions, according to Mor. Medicaid in most states simply does not pay enough.

Regardless of nursing home ownership, the range of quality is enormous. A minority of nursing homes are foul-smelling, Dickensian hellholes where residents are subjected to indifference or outright cruelty at the hands of those paid to care for them. Mor found that low-income African Americans are most likely to live in these substandard homes. At least 16 percent of nursing homes, according to a 2005 study by the U.S. Government Accountability Office, give such poor care that residents are at real risk of harm.[5] But most nursing homes are clean and well maintained, with decent management and kindhearted staff. Still, we dread them.

In his seminal 1980 work on nursing home policy, *Unloving Care: The Nursing Home Tragedy*, Bruce E. Vladeck, former administrator of the Health Care Financing Administration (now the Centers for Medicare and Medicaid Services), wrote:

> Although the overall quality of nursing homes improved substantially in the preceding decade, there were still, in the United States in 1978, nursing homes with green meat and maggots in the kitchen, narcotics in unlocked cabinets, and disconnected sprinklers in nonfire-resistant structures. The increasingly small proportion of truly horrible nursing homes may be less distressing in the aggregate, though, than the quality of life in the thousands that meet the minimal public standards of adequacy. In these, residents live out the last of their days in an enclosed society without privacy, dignity, or pleasure, subsisting on minimally palatable diets, multiple sedatives, and large doses of television—eventually dying, one suspects, at least partially of boredom.[6]

Twenty-five years later, Vladeck maintains that, sadly, while nursing homes have improved the medical care they deliver, the quality of life remains unchanged for far too many residents. Reflecting on the passage just quoted, he wrote in 2003 that the "existential crisis in nursing home care" remained. "Nursing homes are occupied largely by people who, if they could choose, would choose not to be there; staffed by employees of whom many will leave at the first opportunity; and financed primarily by public officials who resent every penny and feel trapped, without alternatives."[7]

It is this existential crisis—for residents and employees alike—that today's advocates are determined to put right.

A Brief History of a Strange Institution

- Rule 5. Furniture and all articles brought into the Home by the applicants or their friends shall be the property of the Home . . .
- Rule 9. After applicants enter the Home, relations and friends who have placed them in our care cannot interfere with the rules and regulations of the Home . . .
- Rule 11. Applicants being received into the Home must agree to accept location of room assigned them by the Executive Committee, which shall have power to make all necessary changes in the occupancy of all rooms.
- Rule 16. Breakfast will be served at 8:15; dinner at 12:30, and supper at 5:00, with the exception of Sunday when a light supper will be served . . .
- Rule 24. It must be understood that these rules are absolute, and must be obeyed at all times; any violation will result in the removal of the offender from the Home.

    —The Home of the Aged and Orphans of the Baltimore
    Conference at the Methodist Episcopal Church South
    rule book, 1930

How did the modern nursing home evolve? No social workers, health professionals, or advocates—let alone older people themselves—sat around and dreamed up what would be the most humane living arrangement for older people who have diminished physical or mental capacities and no one to help them out at home. Rather, decades of disordered actions by state and federal legislators, entrepreneurs, nonprofit agencies, and, eventually, large corporations produced nursing homes.

Throughout our nation's history, we have as a society shown ourselves uncomfortable with people who can't fend for themselves. An unfortunate byproduct of our romantic attachment to rugged individualism and independence has been our view of old people as a social problem. Unlike many traditions around the globe that honor elders for their wisdom, we struggle with what to do with those who are no longer productive economically. The tension between the common good and public costs dates back two hundred years.

As long as we had a farm-based economy, most families expected—and were able—to care for their elders at home. (Interestingly, a 2005 report by the Pew Research Center found that 56 percent of baby boomers said it is a family responsibility to allow an elderly parent to live in your home.)[8] Older people who had neither family nor the means to hire in-home help depended on charity to survive. Some moved in with families in the community who, for a modest fee, provided room and board. In colonial times, those who were poor, for any reason, were often kept in poorhouses or almshouses, where their basic needs were met. To discourage lazy people from gravitating to these, strict rules made life there unpleasant, such as required uniforms and forced confinement to the institution. Everyone was expected to work to contribute to the operation of the place. As time went on, a motley assortment of social outcasts lived in poorhouses, including alcoholics and petty criminals. As poorhouses multiplied in the 1800s, so did reports of horrible living conditions and mistreatment.

"Let us not forget that the true history of our institutional services (both in hospitals and homes) reflects not noble, charitable and altruistic motives, but rather the efforts of society to isolate and to remove from view the diseased and handicapped. The almshouse of the past was the community collection pot for the orphaned, lame, sick, blind, deaf, aged and ofttimes the insane," wrote Herbert Shore, past president of the American Association of Homes for the Aging, in 1966.[9]

Eventually, those who were poor were divided into "the deserving" (the very young and very old) and "the undeserving" (alcoholics and generally shiftless folks). Children were moved into orphanages, those with mental illness into asylums, the undeserving into workhouses. That left elderly people in their own poorhouses—except for those with dementia, who were often lumped with mentally ill people in asylums.

In the late 1800s, immigrant groups and wealthy benefactors created benevolent societies that provided much better accommodations for older, dependent people. But even then, life could be difficult. According to Karen Stevenson, in her history of long-term care, iron-fisted matrons sometimes ran the homes, requiring "inmates" to ask permission to have visitors or to go off the premises.[10]

Meanwhile, in the late nineteenth century, the first hospitals were built. These institutions, too, were typically for poor people—wealthier people could hire in-home help. The old, poor, and ill moved into hospitals for lengthy periods. The Civil War left thousands of disabled veterans who also needed assistance.

Before the twentieth century, eldercare was the responsibility of local communities. But gradually federal and state governments stitched together a patchwork of policies to help old and disabled people. By the Depression, most states had laws requiring children to care for their parents—laws that sometimes were harshly enforced. But the economic disaster had split and impoverished families. The political push during the Depression for old-age assistance thus came less from elderly people themselves than from their families, who could not care for both their children and their aging parents, according to Stevenson.

From its inception in the 1930s, old-age assistance was denied to people living in public almshouses. The goal was to enable people to live in the community, both because it was more dignified than poorhouses and because it was less expensive. By remaining in the community, it was reasoned, old people could still do their modest part to contribute to the running of a household. But many people in institutions were too ill to live in the community. Since public agencies were not allowed to accept old-age assistance funds, for-profit facilities sprang up to fill the gap. "The original entry of for-profit operators into publicly subsidized nursing home services was largely an accident, but with the passage of time, such accidents tend to become irreversible," Vladeck observed.[11]

Small operators, anxious for a new source of income, opened old-age homes by the hundreds. These nursing homes soon developed a bad reputation. Unregulated and unattached to high-quality medical services, for-profit homes often were truly deplorable. In response, in the 1950s, what had been a housing and welfare approach to the "problem" of the elderly shifted to a medical approach.

What followed was a muddled mix of housing and health services. Through the Hill-Burton Act, the federal government in 1954 began providing construction funds to nursing homes that were attached to nonprofit hospitals. Since hospital regulations were already in place, and since the goal was to improve medical care, nonprofit nursing homes followed the hospital model—a well-intentioned measure, but one that led to a poor quality of life for those destined to spend years in such places.

For-profit nursing homes, meanwhile, became eligible for their own pot of federal construction money through the Federal Housing Administration and Small Business Administration. Many operators, including a few with mob connections, got into the business not out of honest concern for older people, but because they saw a lucrative real estate opportunity. Anyone could open a nursing home, no experience required, and some saw a gravy train in what should have been a vital social service. Thousands of nursing homes sprouted throughout the nation, many of them still in operation today.

Well-documented scandals, corruption, and abuse were ongoing. High-profile newspaper accounts, including reports of fires in which dozens of old people were killed, led Congress in 1965, under the leadership of Senator Frank Moss of Utah, to hold hearings on nursing home conditions. Regulations were created to protect the well-being of residents. Today, nursing home operators complain about being "the most regulated industry in America" (recently outpacing even nuclear power in the number of regulations, according to popular report), but the regulations came only after volumes of disgraceful conditions had been exposed.

The passage of Medicare and Medicaid in 1965 further pushed nursing homes toward a medical model. Congress was concerned less with providing a high quality of life for nursing home residents than with protecting the federal budget from an unending drain. Reimbursement was thus tied to specific medical conditions. The many nursing homes constructed as minihospitals, with shared rooms and nurse's stations, adopted a model of care that mirrored life in a hospital.

Medicare and Medicaid did not cover options that would have been more to elders' liking—such as bringing nursing services to their homes or creating other types of congregate or group homes. Many people ended up in a nursing home not so much because they were bedridden or extremely ill, but because they needed help and the government would only pay for that help in a nursing home.

Steve McAlilly, president of Mississippi Methodist Senior Services, explains it this way: "The whole experiment of nursing homes was based on good intentions. People saw what was developing in hospitals—with penicillin, patients got well. The good intentions were to provide good medical care. Then it evolved into a system with Medicaid and Medicare that revolved around efficient treatment rather than quality of life. If we fixed the illness, that must be good. Then it spiraled to what it is today—the customer is not the elder or the family—the customer is the regulator. That's who we're serving."

The New Health Consumer

In the late 1960s and early 1970s, consumer and social justice movements emerged that would help create a climate for nursing home reform. In the medical realm, a patients' rights movement emerged based on reports that people who became active participants in the treatment of their illness, rather than its passive victims, were more likely to survive. The movement helped raise awareness that patients should not be defined or labeled by their disease and called for practitioners to employ a holistic, strengths-based approach to treatment.

Groups such as Ralph Nader's Public Citizen railed against impersonal institutions, the technologizing of health care, and the concern for profits over people. Feminists demanded less-paternalistic treatment by doctors and fought for women to have more control of their health care. The medicalizing of childbirth, intended to prevent maternal and infant mortality, came under attack. The practice of putting women under general anesthesia to give birth in surgical-type delivery rooms, with their infants whisked away to nurseries where the "experts" took over, was challenged. So too was the odd notion, reinforced by formula manufacturers, that bottle feeding was better than breastfeeding. Midwives became licensed, and hospitals introduced homey birthing rooms in the 1980s.

At the other end of the life spectrum, in the late 1960s Dr. Elisabeth Kübler-Ross brought the hospice philosophy, a humane and compassionate approach to dying, from England to the United States. End-of-life, she proposed, was "a final stage of growth," a sacred time of coming to terms with life and saying farewell to loved ones. Modern medicine, she argued, viewed death as a failure that doctors must prevent with every machine and medicine at their disposal. In the 1980s, the government succumbed to years of lobbying and agreed to cover hospice services under Medicare, largely as a cost-cutting measure at the end of life. To this day, far too many dying patients do not take advantage of these comprehensive, holistic services.

Also during this period, muckraker Jessica Mitford went undercover throughout the United States to expose profiteering and manipulation in the funeral business. The book she produced, *An American Way of Death*, documented how bereaved families were skewered by a funeral industry that marketed high-priced embalming, fancy caskets, and an array of extras that cost families thousands of dollars.

Meanwhile, Angelica Thieriot, an ordinary citizen who was hospitalized in 1975 for a life-threatening illness, came away shocked at the impersonal care she received—care that seemed to her the antithesis of healing. She went on to launch Planetree, an organization dedicated to transforming hospitals into person-centered places of healing. The Planetree model advocates empowering patients through education, involving families and friends in the hospital experience, and enriching the sterile environment, among many other changes (see Appendix D). Today's movement to change the culture of nursing homes in many ways mirrors Planetree's patient-centered philosophy.

Also paving the way to new thinking about nursing homes was the movement to deinstitutionalize people with mental retardation and developmental disabilities by providing community-based housing for them.

To the Rescue

Throughout these decades of reform, nursing homes were not immune to public demands for change. Stinging indictments by researchers and journalists appeared, including Vladeck's *Unloving Care*; *Tender Loving Greed* by Mary Adelaid Mendelson; and the Pulitzer Prize-winning *Why Survive? Being Old in America* by gerontologist Robert Butler.

As investigators continued to uncover deplorable conditions in nursing homes, reform advocates grew vocal. In 1975, members of the National Gray Panthers Long-Term Care Action Project organized the National Citizens' Coalition for Nursing Home Reform (NCCNHR), aimed at fighting for higher standards in nursing homes.[12] Early on, the coalition championed not only nursing home residents, but also those who served them. The coalition's first paper, released in 1978, was titled "The Plight of the Nurse Aide in America's Nursing Homes." Over time, the coalition extended its advocacy to small board-and-care homes as well.

NCCNHR, under the passionate leadership of Elma Holder and many other pioneering women, advocated for higher reimbursement, consumer education, and high-quality care. In 1985, the coalition convened small groups of residents in fifteen states—four hundred in all—to speak for themselves on what a high quality of life might mean. Based on these conversations, the coalition released "A Consumer Perspective on Quality Care: The Residents' Point of View." At long last, the voice of elders themselves began to make itself heard.

NCCNHR's efforts got a significant boost in 1986 when the prestigious Institute of Medicine issued a landmark report, "Improving the Quality of Care in Nursing Homes." This in turn led Congress to pass in 1987 the far-reaching Nursing Home Reform Law. (In true bureaucratic fashion, the law, passed as part of the Omnibus Budget Reconciliation Act, has ever since been commonly referred to as OBRA '87.)

As nursing home administrator and early maverick David Green recalls: "OBRA was the most radical and influential nursing home legislation ever, because it fundamentally changed the philosophy. Most of my peers at that time were saying, 'Woe is us—the government is doing it to us again, they're making all these expectations, not saying how to go about it and not giving us any money.' And I'm saying, Yes! Because [the government has] no idea how to do it, and what we need to do is change it fundamentally. This is a mental challenge, not a funding issue. OBRA expected us to align all the elements—operational, management, philosophy, organizational design, technology, physical design—to be resident centered."

The Nursing Home Reform Law promised residents important, basic rights such as choice, privacy, dignity, and unlimited access to visitors (see Appendix A). Hard-won by advocates and enlightened health professionals, the legislation was intended to transform nursing homes by making residents' wishes, rather than institutional efficiency, the highest priority. The goal: facilities that felt as much like "home" as possible.

Meanwhile, beyond Washington, D.C., a handful of progressive nonprofit nursing homes quietly put in place new, more compassionate ways to house and care for people. As far back as 1973, Kendal, a Quaker-based organization in Pennsylvania, established a new kind of retirement community, one that honored the dignity of the individual, no matter how ill or frail. "Their whole philosophy was one of giving people independence and supporting them with their own decision making," said Beryl Goldman, Kendal director of outreach.

Both Kendal, as a provider, and NCCNHR, as an advocacy organization, tackled one of the most disturbing aspects of nursing home life: the physical restraint of residents, either by tying them to furniture or by drugging them. Not a band of sadists but well-intentioned medical professionals supported this practice, convinced that the indignity of restraints was a minor annoyance compared to the risk of residents falling, breaking bones, or disturbing others. (For more on the problems of restraints, see Chapter 3.) To its credit, from the day it opened its doors, Kendal refused to use restraints. It went on to launch the Untie the Elderly campaign to advocate restraint-free environments in nursing homes.

In 1987, reform leader Carter Catlett Williams crossed the ocean to Graber Nursing Home in Gothenburg, Sweden, to learn how it achieved what Carter, like Kendal, envisioned: restraint-free care. At Graber, Carter saw a way of life she scarcely dared imagine for nursing home residents: a system of individualized care based on a philosophy of respect, normalcy, relationship, and choice. She returned to Graber in 1990 with University of Pennsylvania researchers Neville Strumpf and Lois Evans, who strengthened the case against restraints in the United States. The use of restraints in this country has since declined dramatically, from 50 percent of nursing home residents in 1989 to 6 percent in 2006.[13]

There have been other improvements as well, including the increased use of individualized care plans; reduced levels of dehydration, malnutrition, and pressure sores (bedsores); and less use of antipsychotic drugs. But there is still a long way to go.

Despite the victory of the Nursing Home Reform Law, further—again, unintentional—setbacks were in store for people in nursing homes.

In its wisdom, Congress tinkered with the Medicare system in 1988 and created an incentive for nursing homes to devote their energies to "subacute" services, providing temporary care to those discharged from hospitals but needing further rehabilitation. The government paid nursing homes a higher rate to care for these patients, thus reinforcing the very medical model that the reform law had intended to change. "While the growth of subacute services in nursing homes provided enormous benefits to facility proprietors, its benefits to [short-term] nursing home patients or [long-term] residents are much more difficult to identify," notes Vladeck[14].

In the 1990s nursing home residents were pushed further down the social ladder, no easy feat. As assisted living sprang up and grew at a phenomenal rate, many people who would have moved to nursing homes chose this new option. "We have really found a place for these individuals in assisted living," explained former nursing home administrator Andrew Carle, head of the nation's first assisted-living administration program, at George Mason University in Virginia. "They should be able to live their lives and feel comfortable. We've rejected the way we've approached nursing homes. You won't find five people who are looking forward to a nursing home." In a decade, assisted living would mushroom to thirty-six thousand facilities, outstripping nursing homes by two to one.

Another change came in 1999: The Supreme Court ruled in the Olmstead decision that under the Americans with Disabilities Act, public agencies must offer home- and community-based services, instead of institutionalization, to people with mental disabilities, regardless of age. In theory at least, this opens the way for people with dementia to demand such services, rather than be moved to a nursing home to qualify for Medicaid.

No one regrets these developments. Elders and people with disabilities deserve as much choice as possible. But that still leaves long-term nursing home residents—and employees—stuck in the place of last resort. The message is: Anything but a nursing home. Yet home care and assisted living cannot serve everyone's needs, as 1.6 million nursing home residents can attest. And even though the rate of disability among people over eighty-five is declining—welcome news indeed—the sheer number of aging baby boomers suggests that long-term care is here to stay. What form that care takes depends on what we demand.

Problems Persist

Most of us live in a state of denial, if not outright delusion, about our own prospects for ever needing care. A 2002 survey by the GE Center for Financial Learning found that 85 percent of adults in the United States who live independently thought they would never need long-term care, such as home-health services or a nursing home. A 2004 MetLife Mature Market Institute poll found that a laughable 14 percent of baby boomers anticipated they would ever need day-to-day assistance. Yet predictions are that *50 to 70 percent* of Americans will need some sort of long-term care.[15]

This does not come as good news to most of us, of course. A 2005 Kaiser Family Foundation public opinion survey found that only 35 percent thought nursing homes do a "good job."[16] Nursing homes ranked lower in this regard than did nurses, doctors, and hospitals—lower even than pharmaceutical companies and barely above insurance companies.

The nursing home "industry," as it unfortunately calls itself, insists that the news media are to blame for the public's dread. The industry claims that the press hypes problems, while ignoring improvements.

But in the Kaiser survey, respondents weren't basing their negative views on media horror stories: 84 percent had some experience with nursing homes, either as a visitor or a resident. Nearly half had a family member or close friend in a nursing home in the previous three years. Forty-one percent thought people actually get worse in a nursing home, while only 19 percent thought they were better off.

It's safe to say that none of the people who end up in a nursing home believed, when they were younger, they would spend the end of their days in the monochrome, slow-motion world of an institution. But many of us—millions of us—will.

Our denial springs not only from our fear of being incapacitated. We probably feel we could bear the discomforts of illness or disability if we were cared for at home by loved ones or by kindly, paid caregivers. Our fear has less to do with our actual physical decline than with the nursing home institution itself and its attendant loss of control, privacy, intimacy, and joy. "Nursing homes are purgatory," English professor Joyce Horner wrote in her remarkable chronicle of her three-year residency in one.[17]

Although meaningful advances have been made, plenty of fuel remains to stoke continuing criticism. According to state long-term care ombudsman data, from 1996 through 2000, the number of nursing home complaints increased from 145,000 to 186,000. This represented a 28 percent increase in the number of complaints and a 30 percent increase in the number of complaints per thousand beds.[18] The top six complaint categories: Failure to respond to call lights or requests for assistance, accidents and improper handling of residents, lack of adequate care plans and resident assessments, inadequate administration of medications, unattended resident symptoms, and poor personal hygiene—not exactly frivolous concerns. The number of reported abuse cases rose from 13,469 in 1996 to 15,501 in 1998, then dropped a bit to 15,010 in 2000, with physical abuse the most common type reported. The ombudsmen believe that complaints are significantly underreported.

A single issue of the *AARP Bulletin* (September 2004) included four articles related to shoddy nursing home practices:

- One told the story of a maverick pharmacist, Armon B. Neel, Jr., whose mission was to halt the overmedication of older people. He maintained that 80 percent of long-term care residents are overmedicated and that most could cut their medication levels in half. The result would be "fewer hospital stays, fewer hospital admissions, lower labor costs involved in care, and a better quality of life for residents," he said.
- A news brief noted that 30 percent of nursing homes still do not have sprinklers for fire safety.
- Another article told of Melville Borne, Jr., who owned three nursing homes in Louisiana that often had inadequate supplies of soap, bandages, and disinfectants. The sheets were "so threadbare that they resembled netting." Meanwhile, Borne had a 150-acre riverfront estate, a corporate plane, and an annual salary of $250,000. The story's headline suggested a suitable punishment: Send him to a nursing home.
- Perhaps the worst report described an undercover investigation by the State of New Mexico. Trained agents posed as nursing home residents in three homes with a poor record of care. Chris Christensen pretended he had Alzheimer's disease and spent five days in a nursing home, where he was greeted by smiling staff members who promised his stay would be just like a "hotel." Unable to stomach the meals of "gray, liquidy pancake" and "canned stew," he lost ten pounds. No one helped residents, their fingers bent with arthritis, as they struggled to open packets of saltines. Water pitchers sat empty for days. Other undercover agents had even worse tales to tell, of urine-stained sheets and filthy bathrooms.

In response to this piece, an AARP member wrote to the editor about his own dismal experience in an Ohio nursing home. "I spent 10 weeks in a nursing home after I broke both wrists. The mental abuse, degradation and lack of attention often go unobserved by the casual visitor. Aides, nurses, and administrative staff often overlook or ignore residents' concerns. . . . As a 57-year-old baby boomer, I had the opportunity to glimpse the future, and it is not pleasant."

In fact, had it not been for investigations by the press and the government, prompted by reform advocates, nursing homes would be far worse than they are today. Regulations, surveys, fines, and even prison sentences forced many nursing home administrators to clean up their act or go out of business. But even giving nursing home providers the benefit of the doubt—that they are misunderstood—we have a problem. As Joani Latimer, state long-term care ombudsman for Virginia put it: "The current system, on the best days in the best places with the best intentions, is still so far from how I think we should define life in our final years."

Putting Elders Out to Pasture

Nursing homes are a predictable outgrowth of a U.S. culture that views old age as a disease to be prevented or conquered, rather than a life stage to be honored. We have long segregated those who are very old or ill, treating them as expendable to community life. As a society, we set them out on the ice floe, wish them luck, and get on with the important business of living.

"Collectively, old age is, at least in American culture, generally negatively valued as a time of loss of social roles and physical vigor and, consequently of increased dependency," write researchers Robert L. Rubinstein and Patricia A. Parmelee.[19]

These views are beginning to change, at least regarding healthy, active older people. But we often marginalize those who are frail, ill, or the "oldest old."

A "Dear Abby" column a few years back was illustrative.[20] "Undecided in St. Paul" was planning a wedding. The problem: whether or not to invite a relative who lived in a nursing home. "Undecided" didn't want the relative to feel obligated to send a gift. That the relative might actually want to attend was not considered. Abby suggested that in lieu of an invitation, the family send a chatty letter after the fact so that the relative could remain "in the loop."

No doubt the advice maven herself would have felt angry and hurt to receive a letter from a relative describing what fun everyone had at a wedding to which she had not been invited.

Readers let her have it. One nurse who worked in a nursing home wrote that residents should be included in important family events: "If friends and family only knew how these people felt sitting in their rooms or in hallways with nothing to do." Another reader opined: "Send the invitation! Better to be engaged in life than disengaged. I want to make my own decisions, don't you?"

To her credit—and perhaps her humility is one reason why readers were so loyal to Abby—the columnist admitted she'd been wrong. "I should pay less attention to my brain and more attention to what my heart tells me," she wrote in a mea culpa.

Most of us have such moments, when we close our hearts and allow ourselves to view those in nursing homes as somehow not like us—at least until it is our own mother or father, or we ourselves, who lives in one. Nursing home residents are not just old, an attribute little valued in our culture, but they are ill. We treat them as has-beens who contribute nothing and who take up space until they die. In his book *In the Shadow of Memory*, Floyd Skloot reflects on how it feels to be impaired by illness—in his case, brain damage suffered as the result of a bizarre virus. "Removed from the customary worlds of calendar and clock time, the obligations of work, the fields of play, a chronically ill person seems to have stumbled, to be out of sync," he writes. "Such people are often viewed as a counterweight, pulling the economy down with them, creating a burden on those who still work."[21]

Of course we wish people in nursing homes no harm, and we want them safe and well cared for. But we don't really believe they are capable of living fully and enjoying day-to-day pleasures that we take for granted. They are slumpers.

When I began exploring this topic, I toured a church-affiliated nursing home in Washington, D.C., that is considered one of the best in the city. The chipper social worker who escorted me was nice enough. With short hair and dressed in navy sweatpants and white polo shirt, she reminded me of a high school gym coach.

She showed me the sparkling swimming pool, the lovely chapel, the dining hall—everything clean and orderly. When I asked to see the residents' quarters, she took me to a room she thought was uninhabited. As she began to explain the room's amenities, we heard the person in the adjoining space groan loudly. The social worker looked embarrassed and muttered something like, "Oh, great." Hearing our voices, the woman moaned again.

The response of the social worker was dispiriting: She did nothing. She didn't ask the woman what was the matter or murmur reassuringly to her. Instead, she hurriedly led me, her silent accomplice, from the room. As we left the wing, she told no one on the staff that the woman down the hall might need assistance. We continued the tour, but for me the place had lost its luster.

The incident spoke volumes about the attitude of this and so many nursing homes. Efficiency reigned. It was the end of the day, the social worker wanted to finish up, perhaps the woman moaned a lot. Then again, perhaps she moaned because she knew we were there, and she assumed we would hear her and inquire what she needed. I blame myself as well. I could have asked the woman if she needed help—or at least asked the social worker how we should respond. The fact that we both ignored the moaning meant that we saw the sufferer as someone not like us.

Moaning, I have since learned, is not simply irritating background noise, like Muzak in the elevator. Moaning is a call for help. It could mean something as simple as wanting a glass of water, or it could be something as awful as having untreated pain or desperately needing to go to the bathroom. Or it could come out of sheer loneliness or the futility of life. But it is not normal, even in the context of a nursing home, nor is it normal to ignore it—any more than it would be normal if you were lying on the couch, moaning, and a friend—or in this case, a stranger—entered your house and walked right by you.

We need to rethink the significance of a woman alone in her room, moaning. She could be our mother—or she could be us. We need to reclaim her as a vital part of our tribe.

To do this requires fundamentally transforming both the culture of nursing homes and our societal attitudes. People who have lived long have rich experience from which we can learn. They are vital human beings who take pleasure in everyday life and in having close relationships. They want opportunities to tell their life stories or simply to enjoy looking at the sky, petting a cat, cracking a joke, or listening to music. The idea of elders as respected members of the community must be reclaimed and reshaped for the modern world.

At an excellent retirement community in the Midwest, I met a couple who confided that they feared nothing more than being moved to the nursing home wing. They had plotted a contingency. They owned a cabin on a small piece of land. If one of them began to fail, they planned to escape there. Better to go without medical care, they reasoned, than to be caught in the web of the nursing home.

That the traditional culture of these institutions inspires such fear and dread in older people should certainly give us pause. Is there no better way?

In fact, there is. Across the country, under the radar, a quiet revolution has been percolating. Independent of one another, enlightened people leading nursing homes have been experimenting with a new concept of care. In 1995, at its annual conference, NCCNHR convened a panel of these visionaries—Charlene Boyd; Bill Thomas, MD.; Barry Barkan; and Joanne Rader—whom Carter Williams had met through her efforts to ban restraints. The panelists had not collaborated before, yet they held strikingly similar philosophies, each under a different label: resident-directed care, the Eden Alternative, the regenerative community, individualized care.

After that first meeting, a second gathering of thirty-three selected leaders was held in Rochester in 1997. This is how Karen Schoeneman, senior policy analyst with the Centers for Medicare and Medicaid Services Division of Nursing Homes, recalls it:

> There was a horrible blizzard. Our plane couldn't land in Rochester. They landed in Buffalo and we went by taxi for forty miles on really slippery roads. . . . They had invited mostly people from the business, one researcher, me, and a couple from state government who they really trusted. They wanted to get the people together who 'got it.' And what a group they got together! They had us in session, in dialogue with each other, from breakfast until ten o'clock at night. We slept together dormitory style. And by the end of that time, we had started a movement.

They went on to create a coalition, the Pioneer Network, dedicated to transforming the culture of nursing homes. "We're not talking about innovation," said Carter Williams. "We're talking about deep philosophical and systems change. We also aim to change the culture of aging in this country."

The pioneers were soon joined by others, such as Steve Shields of Meadowlark Hills in Kansas and Eric Haider, then at Crestview Nursing Home in Missouri.

"The Pioneer movement is what gives us hope that care can be better in this country, because we see care, both quality of life and quality of care, in these facilities that's just superb," said Alice H. Hedt, executive director of NCCNHR. "So it gives us a vision that we know can be achieved."

The Pioneer Network began from the point of shared values, rather than an intent to tinker with cost containment, regulations, or federal policies. From these values, they are discerning what people in nursing homes need and want, explained Carter. "I don't know what the setting will be—but most of us feel very strongly that it's unlikely that we'll continue with the big institutions, because they're deadening places to live in and work in. And we need life, not death," she said.

Across the nation, from Tupelo, Mississippi, to Seattle, Washington; Manhattan, Kansas, to Rochester, New York, I have witnessed profound change inside nursing homes. Culture-change leaders are tearing up everything—the floor plans, the flow charts, the schedules, the lousy menus, the attitudes, the rules—and starting from scratch. They are creating extraordinary places where people live in dignity and greet the day with contentment, assisted by employees who feel valued and appreciated. Perhaps most surprising, these homes prove that a high quality of life does not have to cost more. Some of the best homes in the nation serve primarily low-income people who are on Medicaid.

The following chapters tell the story of a better way to live in old age. Although each home is different, they share common values: honoring individual choices; empowering staff; fostering a strong community of elders, staff, family members, and volunteers; redesigning buildings from a hospital model to a home; breaking down barriers with the outside world; maintaining a sense of purpose and meaning; and honoring people when they die.

Whether these transformational homes become the norm or the domain of a lucky few is the question that faces the next generation of elders, the baby boomers. Many forces are aligned to bring about fundamental change in our societal view of aging. But tremendous hurdles remain. Those on the front lines today demonstrate that change in the most intractable setting, the nursing home, is possible—painstaking and laborious, but possible. Whether we believe it is worth the trouble is up to us.

"If [nursing home residents] have a physical or mental problem, it doesn't mean they have lost who they were," said administrator Eric Haider. "They are good citizens. They have worked hard in their life for us. They built this country. They fought in the wars. They've done so much for us, and now they're in the nursing home. It's our job to give them the best—not by bossing them around, but by simply asking them what they want, how they want it, listening to them, honoring their desires. It's a very simple concept: give them what they want."[22]

Chapter 2

"I Almost Cried"

The Universal Longing for Home

Domestic well-being is a fundamental human need that is
deeply rooted in us, and that must be satisfied.
—Witold Rybczynski, *Home: A Short History of an Idea*

What is the matter with us that when you need home the
most—when you need community the most, when you need
choice the most, when you need self-confidence the most,
when you need relationships the most—you don't have it.
It never even occurred to us that where you live could be a
home.
—Steve Shields, nursing home administrator

In the spring of 1999, Steve Shields, administrator of a well-regarded nursing home in Manhattan, Kansas, was in the midst of an upheaval of his own making. Convinced that the organization he led was stagnating, he had embarked on an ambitious campaign to transform Meadowlark Hills.

His plan was going well. He had persuaded a smaller nursing home in the community to close its doors and merge with his own, as a way to make both more financially stable. He had led one of the largest fund-raising campaigns ever seen in Manhattan, garnering $3.5 million in donations and a $30 million bond. Renovations were under way to modernize and spruce up the nursing home. The staff mood over the proposed changes ranged from hostile to enthusiastic. But things were moving forward.

Still, something was not right.

A friendly Midwesterner, Steve is an optimist. He may be the only nursing home administrator in the world whose former career was in offshore oil drilling. Accustomed to seeing clearly the path to solving problems, this time Steve felt a nagging sense of unease about the changes under way at Meadowlark Hills. Everything he had envisioned was coming to pass, but he took no joy in it.

> Construction trailers were on site, framing was up, we were roofing and I got this pit in my stomach. It was there for two months. I thought I had an ulcer. I couldn't get rid of that pit. And the pit was telling me, "You're off. You're not doing the right thing." I'm thinking, three-and-a-half million dollars that we've gone to the community for, we've got investors, we're going to close this facility across town, and you're telling me I'm doing the wrong thing! But I couldn't ignore it.

Unable to determine what was wrong, he convened a gathering of consultants in organizational change. They flew in from around the country. Steve sat them down in a circle, inviting them to give their pitch. They all seemed cut from the same mold: well-dressed glad-handers with slick proposals, versed in "pulling in stakeholders" and "posturing the organization." All of them, except one. She was a middle-aged woman from Milwaukee, with strong features, large tortoise-shell glasses, and auburn hair pulled back in a French twist. She seemed more down-to-earth than the others, quiet but determined. When her turn came to speak, she leaned forward, looked him in the eye, and said: "You need to put the resident in the driver's seat, and you need to create teams that will empower the residents in such a way that they will continue the fabric of their lives." Then she sat back, letting her words sink in.

That was LaVrene Norton. Steve soon bade the others farewell, and he and LaVrene talked for hours. Before she left, she told him he must make a journey. "There's a place you have to see up in Bigfork, Minnesota," she told him.

Yeah, right, he thought. I can't even see my desk or return phone calls, I've got so much work to do. I'm heading up this major construction project that I know nothing about. There's no way I'm leaving town now. "Maybe in two or three months," he told her.

But she insisted that he go immediately. In fact, she intimated, he should have gone months ago.

So he put his faith in her. He and his two directors of nursing drove two hours to Kansas City, flew to Minneapolis, took a puddle jumper to Grand Rapids, Minnesota, and spent the night in a lodge next to Judy Garland's childhood home—something he would later find symbolic.

Early the next morning, they rented a car and drove forty miles up the two-lane Edge of the Wilderness Highway, past small ponds and stands of birch, to Bigfork, population ninety-eight. Following the blue hospital signs, they finally reach their destination. Steve didn't know what he was expecting—some kind of Shangri-La for elders, something architecturally stunning, perhaps.

But the modest brick structure looked like every 1960s-era nursing home he'd ever seen. "I pull up and I'm thinking, 'LaVrene! Damn it! I caught a puddle jumper and drove all the way up here for this?' It was this little tiny place, and it looked like it hadn't been updated since the Medicare Act."

When they entered the facility, they were met by administrator Linda Bump. She was a short, fast-talking woman who was warm and friendly, but clearly on a mission. She launched into a rapid-fire spiel about her philosophy of "resident-centered care." "I'm thinking, 'This woman's crazy,'" said Steve. "'I like her.'"

Bigfork Valley Communities (formerly Northern Pines) could not afford to renovate its entire building, Bump explained. She showed them first the old wing of the nursing home: long hallways, double rooms, a nurse's station. Steve felt his impatience returning.

But then it happened. She led them to the new section, Spruce Lodge. Steve saw a nursing home like none he had ever imagined. "We walked in the door, and that feeling in my stomach—it was gone. I swear to God. I walked in there, and it was like I had a physical sensation. This is it. It crystallized everything for me. Everything came into completely clear focus. I almost cried."

Home as Sacred Space

What Steve Shields recognized in that moment was "home." He saw it in a deeply familiar way, as you would if you visited your favorite aunt. You would ring the doorbell before entering, and she would invite you in. On the mantle would be family photos, on the bookshelves would be her worn copies of Shakespeare or the Bible. The cushions on the couch would be contoured to her body. She would go to the kitchen and pour you a glass of sweet tea or port, urging you to sit down. The dwelling, no matter how humble, would be her domain.

Until Steve walked into Spruce Lodge, he had never imagined that this comfortable sense of home could exist behind the walls of a nursing facility.

That this recognition was enough to make a take-charge guy get weepy says as much about the typical nursing home as it does about Bigfork. Nursing homes, as we know, are far from homey. As researchers Rubinstein and

Parmelee observed: "The majority of modern nursing homes and other long-term care facilities are 'nonplaces' that afford no links with one's personal or cultural past" and promote "social roles such as 'old' and 'sick.'"[1]

The "home" in most nursing homes is more marketing myth than reality. Home, like the air we breathe, is something that most of us take for granted. What makes a home? The obvious answer is that home is where we live—yet not every place we live is home. According to *Webster's New World Dictionary*, home is "a place where one likes to be; restful or congenial place; the place that is the natural environment of an animal, plant, etc."

Restful, congenial, natural. From a biological standpoint, a natural environment is the ecosystem in which organisms evolved and continue to thrive. The very word "ecosystem" is wrapped up with home: *eco*, from the Greek *oikos*, meaning house or dwelling.

The longing for home is woven into the genetic makeup of many species. Anthropologist Loren Eiseley, in his moving essay "The Brown Wasps," writes: "We cling to a time and a place because without them man is lost, not only man but life. . . . This feeling runs deep in life; it brings stray cats running over endless miles, and birds homing from the ends of the earth."[2]

At its most basic level, home for *Homo sapiens* is a place with sufficient food and water, with shelter from the elements. But home is more than that. Humans are social animals. We evolved among, and depend upon, a community of family, friends, and neighbors. Our homes are separate, giving us autonomy and privacy, yet clustered together; even humans who live as nomads move together, so that for them "home" is literally the community and its belongings.

The longing for home reverberates through the world's great stories, from the Homeric epics to Huck Finn, *The Wizard of Oz*, and *The Lord of the Rings*. The narrative of separation from home, initiation, and return to home echoes throughout history and cultures, according to Joseph Campbell in *The Hero with a Thousand Faces*. Heroes have adventures, slay the dragons, gain power or wisdom, but in the end, they head for home.

All of us understand the magnetic pull of home in a visceral way.

In the summer of 2003, social justice activists in a Catholic parish in Cleveland invited homeless women, most of them African American, and middle-class women, most of them white from a well-to-do suburb, to sit down together and talk about what home meant to them. The exercise was a warm-up for the women, who were preparing to lobby their members of Congress on the need for affordable housing.

Each participant received a sheet of paper on which was drawn a simple outline of a house. They were asked to write in the house phrases that captured what home meant to them. They then shared what they'd written. The answers from these two groups of women of different class and race were nearly identical, said Anne Curtis, a Sister of Mercy, who led the meeting. Home, according to the participants, is a place that is affordable, safe, secure, and clean. Home has enough space not to be crowded, with a yard and trees. Home gives us privacy, is free from discrimination, and is peaceful, loving, worry free, and welcoming; a sacred space; a place where I can be myself.

That same year, at the Village, a Methodist retirement community in Indianola, Iowa, residents and staff participated in a similar exercise. The Village, like Meadowlark Hills, is a "continuing care retirement community" that offers a spectrum of living options, from independent townhouses and apartments to assisted-living studios and nursing home rooms. The Village was beginning a major transformation, much like the one Steve Shields was to lead.

At a gathering led by LaVrene Norton, a group of residents and staff talked about the changes they would like to see in the nursing home. LaVrene explained how most nursing homes are based on a hospital model. "The goal is to move to a social model," she said. "This is in line with what people feel in their hearts. What we want for ourselves and our loved ones is home."

She invited participants, seated at small tables, to contrast how life in a medical institution differs from that in our own homes. They then shared their ideas with the full group. Said one older resident, to general laughter, "In the hospital you can't choose your cell mates, and in your home, visitors don't have to sit on the bed."

"In the hospital," offered another, "modesty and privacy are ignored."

"Visitors are restricted—when they come and who they are."

"At home, you take a bath in privacy, when you feel like it."

"We all have bad habits—at home we're allowed to."

"Home is less inhibiting—if you're unhappy, you can yell!"

As these comments suggest and writers elsewhere have observed, nursing homes do not resemble home so much as the "total institutions" Erving Goffman describes in his 1961 classic sociological book, *Asylums*.[3] Total institutions, including prisons, mental hospitals, boot camps, boarding schools, and "old folk's homes," are confined settings where "inmates" must sleep, play, and work. All aspects of their lives take place under one roof, managed by a single authority. All are treated the same and required to do similar activities together in a tightly scheduled routine, "the whole sequence of activities being imposed from above by a system of explicit formal rulings and a body of officials," wrote Goffman. Daily life is planned so as to fulfill the goals of the institution, rather than the desires of the individual.

Despite the Nursing Home Reform Law's promise, the primacy of the institution remains endemic in nursing homes. Whether you are a lifelong opera lover, avid gardener, sports nut, or gourmet cook is irrelevant to overworked, harried staff. You are told when and what to eat. No matter that you have been a lifelong night owl, your bedtime will be eight o'clock, and you will be rousted at dawn. If you enjoyed long, lingering bubble baths after dinner, you will be disappointed. You will be assigned a time and day to be bathed, and, covered only with a sheet, you may be taken down a long hall to the shower room when it is your turn. Privacy is a thing of the past, as you will likely have a roommate and unannounced intrusions by employees. Activities listed on the calendar—bingo, old-time music, holiday crafts—may feel more like busywork than like meaningful or enjoyable pastimes. You are isolated from the wider world, isolated even from others in a retirement community such as the Village or Meadowlark Hills.

Visitors to a nursing home typically enter through a lobby that is hushed and artificial feeling—more like a motel lobby than a living room. A receptionist will ask your business and direct you to a wing of resident bedrooms. Professional staff who reign from behind a nurse's station—the seat of power—oversee each wing. Charts, doctor's orders, care plans, are reserved for the professionals; the direct care—helping residents dress, eat, go to the bathroom, bathe—rests in the hands of underpaid aides who are told what to do and excluded from the inner sanctum of decision making.

In front of the nurse's station, a regular coterie of residents often clusters in wheelchairs, like a flock of birds hoping for crumbs of conversation or activity. A few are alert; others are propped up or slump in various postures of debility or defeat, often too drugged or discouraged to hope even for a crumb. Others roam the halls with no apparent purpose or destination.

One of the most irritating things you notice may be the noise—various chimes or beeps of alarms signaling a call light or someone on "falls prevention" trying to stand or escape. Disembodied voices over the loudspeaker call for staff. Often, residents moan loudly or yell incoherently.

Crowding the hallways are large carts with meal trays, medications, linens, or cleaning supplies. In the worst facilities, the air smells fetid.

Stroll down the hall, and you can't help glancing nosily into residents' rooms. Most residents have to share a room with a stranger with whom they may or may not get along. It might be the middle of the afternoon, but some may still be in their pajamas, watching TV, napping, the leaden routine broken only by meals at regimented times, the assigned bath, or the occasional visitor. The lucky ones regularly see devoted family members. But many are not so fortunate.

Bill Thomas has identified what he calls "the three plagues" rampant in even the best traditional nursing homes: loneliness, helplessness, and boredom. Opportunities are minimal for elders to care for others, to grow, to plan or partake in normal activities.

The very language of the nursing home is institutional and impersonal.

As architect Witold Rybczynski writes: "Words are important. Language is not just a medium, like a water pipe, it is a reflection of how we think."[4]

Language serves to obfuscate the institution. Some long-term care facilities, for example, market life there as one big joyride on a cruise ship. In his book *Nobody's Home: Candid Reflections of a Nursing Home Aide*, Tom Gass writes of the dismal place where he worked: "One of our nursing home brochures invites potential customers to 'imagine yourself in a fine resort.' Come on. This is not a vacation spot. We are a business, and businesses are designed to make money. . . . We expect salespeople to put the best spin on the facts, but we at the front know that our stock-in-trade is human misfortune."[5]

Other nursing homes use language in a way that distances, depersonalizes, or infantilizes those who live there. In fact, many companies no longer bother to use the word "home." The administrator where Gass worked insisted, "It's not a home. It's a nursing facility."[6] Other chains use terms such as "long-term hospitals." (Can you imagine saying, "It's time you go to the long-term hospital, Mom"?) People don't "move" to a nursing home, they are "admitted." Once there, they become patients or even "beds," as when aides are assigned beds or rooms rather than people. Administrators do not visit with residents, they "work the floor." You are labeled by your diagnosis, as the "hip" or "the Parkinson's" in room 278. You switch from living to "having a care plan." You are measured by the number of ADLs (activities of daily living) in which you are deficient or by your MDS (Minimum Data Set), a clinical assessment tool. If you have trouble swallowing and need help eating, you are a "feeder." You may wear a "bib" at mealtime or "diapers" if you are incontinent. If the staff are benevolent, they will "allow" you to make a few choices about your daily life, such as what to wear. But the primary emphasis is medical, custodial, and negative. Life revolves around what you can't do: walk, go to the bathroom by yourself, bathe, get dressed, go outside alone, shop, escape.

Imagine how that would feel, said LaVrene Norton. Imagine moving to this, your new "home." Casting herself in that role, she asks in horror: "You mean my physical problems are *all* we're going to focus on the rest of my life?"

Freeing the Inmates

People who must move to a nursing home, or even to an assisted-living apartment, give up a lot. They have already faced tremendous loss—perhaps the death of a spouse or beloved siblings and friends, the ability to drive, and some of their mental or physical abilities. They often are wrenched away from their church, neighborhood, and other social networks. A friend of mine who is ninety-two years old recently moved to a faith-based assisted-living center and was dismayed to find she was not free to sit where she pleases in the dining room.

Many women I met moved straight to the nursing home from a hospital after a medical crisis without ever returning home. To pay for their care, relatives had to sell these women's homes for them and distribute the contents. To demonstrate how such loss would feel, LaVrene Norton led a group of staff and independent residents at the Village in a simple exercise in which I participated.

LaVrene told us to write down a list of things related to our home that were most precious to us. My list included such things as our front porch, where I sit and listen to birds and chat with neighbors; the kitchen where I cook for family and friends; and my jungle of houseplants. LaVrene then told us to imagine we had to move to a nursing home. One by one, in the order we would choose, we crossed off our list what we would not be allowed to keep. I had to cross off everything on my list. I was taken aback by how painful this little exercise was. When I got to the final item on my list—our beloved Labrador, Ella—I got tears in my eyes.

What does it mean, psychologically, emotionally, to suddenly have no genuine home—especially if you are at your most vulnerable?

In *The Nursing Home in American Society*, researchers Colleen L. Johnson and Leslie A. Grant wrote that the loss of privacy, sense of self, and personal autonomy, along with segregation from the outside world, have serious ill effects on nursing home residents, including "decreased psychological functioning, disengagement from social relationships, and a higher risk of mortality."[7]

Psychiatrist Mindy Thompson Fullilove of Columbia University has examined the importance of a sense of place to health and well-being. Studies of refugees, disaster victims, and residents of neighborhoods destroyed by urban renewal projects suggest that people are deeply traumatized by their loss of home. "Individuals strive for a sense of belonging to a place," she writes. "This sense of belonging arises from the operation of three psychological processes: familiarity, attachment, and identity. Displacement ruptures these emotional connections. The ensuing disorientation, nostalgia, and alienation may undermine the sense of belonging, in particular, and mental health, in general."[8] In other words, losing your home can have serious psychological and emotional consequences.

Older people, especially, may be stressed and anxious when they are uprooted. In fact, the very move that is meant to provide them with better care may actually worsen their medical and emotional problems, according to numerous studies. The institution itself introduces a new set of potential problems, such as infections and bedsores.

Nursing homes may trigger agitation, depression, and submissiveness in residents. As with other confined groups, nursing home residents often exhibit "deindividuation," growing more dependent and less competent and assertive. "One is forced to accept the authority of the staff and thus lose the capacity for controlling one's environment. In the process, the ability to make decisions is affected. As deindividuation proceeds, individual differences among residents are less noticeable, and an impression of sameness among the residents is observable," according to Johnson and Grant.[9]

In a 1992 study of the institutionalized elderly published in the *Journal of Gerontological Nursing*, Judith T. Carboni found that the experience of nursing home residents closely resembled that of homeless people.[10] Among the shared feelings: helplessness, dependency, lack of choices, loss of identity, uprootedness, not belonging, loss of place, vulnerability, intrusion by others, and retreat to an inner world. Is it any wonder that nearly half of nursing home residents are diagnosed with depression? Indeed, it is surprising that this figure is not higher.

Many people, including family members, believe that nursing home residents are slumped over not out of resignation about their fate but out of physical impairment. I learned how deeply held this belief can be when I took a writers' workshop where we each presented our book proposals. After I summarized the major themes of this book, another participant spoke up. Smiling grimly, she told the group that her own father was in a nursing home, and she knew of what she spoke. People in nursing homes are incapable of appreciating life anymore. They are far too ill. Laughter? Helping take care of a Chihuahua or a cockatiel? Engaging with children? Going to the state fair? Not possible. Clearly, she indicated, it was a mistake for me to write a book that would give readers hope.

She is not the only person I have encountered who believes that nursing home residents are too far gone to enjoy a dignified, high-quality life. As Tom Kitwood writes in *Dementia Reconsidered*: "Beliefs, when backed up by accepted authority, acquire a kind of self-evident quality, and are transmuted into the unassailable verities of common sense."[11]

But there is another side of the story. Many—perhaps most—nursing home residents are not as far gone as they appear. Some may live at a pace that to us seems impossibly slow. They may be too deaf, too forgetful, too confused, too much in pain, too exhausted, to readily respond. A woman I met at Meadowlark Hills, for example, appeared at first to be a "slumper." But when I sat down next to her and talked, she was friendly and sweet, inviting me to come see her room. Skilled and loving caregivers have taught me that the key to being present for people with diminished capabilities is to slow down and get into their rhythm, rather than try to force them into ours.

Christa Hojlo, director of Veterans Administration nursing home care, reflected on why she became committed to cultural transformation. She is familiar with the refrain that residents are "too far gone."

> I hear all the time, "All you're saying about nursing home care is really great, but what about the guy with profound dementia that does nothing but wander around all day and is totally disconnected, and what about the guy who needs chemo—we have to apply the medical model." My response is, nursing home folks need medical care, but it has to be a model focused by nurturance, comfort, and love. We do take care of people who have complex chronic medical problems, and people with profound dementias, and those who are dying. That is all the more reason to provide an environment of care that is bright, has good lighting, that invites them to their fullest capacity. [If you are ill], it doesn't mean you can't sit up in bed and enjoy a view outdoors, guided by somebody. It doesn't mean you can't be helped into a chair and brought into the dining room, just because you have tubes. The environment itself and our interactions need to send messages to people, regardless of why they are there, in whatever condition they are in, that we will provide them whatever they need to help them see beyond being a sick person—not that you'll make them well, but there are opportunities to touch the spirit. Our nursing homes should not look like hospitals or feel like hospitals. They should be about gentle interactions.

Christa is now leading a nationwide transformation of VA nursing homes.

Culture-change leaders such as Christa Hojlo, Steve Shields, and Bill Thomas maintain that nursing homes themselves accelerate decline and nudge their residents into apathy, lethargy, and confusion. Deinstitutionalizing the environment and recreating a sense of home can encourage them instead to continue to grow, to learn, to take pleasure in life, to remain engaged. Their infirmities do not disappear, but their illness does not define their lives.

"We have an intrinsic need for a home—our dreams are around it," said Steve Shields. "They're pretty central to us. Why, when you need one the most, do you suddenly not have one? Wherever you reside and live has to be home. Period. It's a basic fundamental flaw in our planning for people with special needs—we don't expect them to be home. So they become wards and responsibilities. We dehumanize them."

No one sets out to inflict these calamities on our elders. We are unable to care for them, and we seek help from those trained to do so. They in turn do the best that they can, given the limited resources and seemingly limitless rules to which they must adhere. The problem is the system itself, which was established not to be homey but to provide medical care as efficiently as possible. A 2002 editorial in the *Journal of Gerontology* noted regretfully the policy decisions to "medicalize the nursing home industry." While improved medical care was the result, the editors observed, "it has also been associated with increased bureaucratic regulations that have decreased the ability of residents to live in a homelike atmosphere for their final years."[12]

"We have an ethical obligation in this country, not just the VA," said Christa Hojlo. "If we're going to save people's lives and help them live into the nineties or one hundreds, we have a responsibility not to dump them, for God's sake. Do we spend megabucks on medications and treatment, just to be warehoused? What are we becoming as a culture? I find it abhorrent. I come to work every day hoping to make a little tiny dent in transforming the social system."

The Elusiveness of Home

Is it realistic to expect a nursing home to be a true home?

Martha Stitelman, MD, a gerontologist in Bennington, Vermont, has worked in a variety of nursing homes for two decades. A practical, no-nonsense New Englander, she brings a healthy skepticism to the question of making deep change in the culture of long-term care. We sat for five hours on a wintry day in downtown Brattleboro, discussing whether fundamental change is possible. "By and large the staff at places I work do care," she said. "There is real affection there. There are not a lot of bedsores or serious falls or medication errors. They are clean and pass the smell test and are in lovely surroundings—and I wouldn't want to live there myself. They are so far from being a place where I would want to live."

I asked her what they would have to become for her to want to live there. "I would have to have a private room, with not only my own furniture, but I would be able to choose my own curtains and paint color," she said. "There would be a sunny window in winter and a tree to sit under in summer—a gazebo is not a tree. There would be no beeping and buzzing. You wouldn't get woken up at night, but there would always be someone to talk to if you couldn't sleep. There would be small areas to read in. To really live there, you wouldn't need a lot of record keeping. I wouldn't take any pills other than for pain. There would be no shoveling of pudding into my mouth."

This doesn't seem too much to ask. I have yet to visit a place, though, that meets all Dr. Stitelman's criteria. Because of regulations, there is not a nursing home in the United States that does not keep voluminous records. And most dispense multiple medications beyond pain pills. But as I will show, many places meet most of Dr. Stitelman's other wishes.

Within our grasp are places where we can feel a sense of belonging, of control to the best of our abilities, of freedom to plan our day, of being in a supportive community. Old age itself is not a barrier to forging attachments to a new home. "One can form any number of bonds with place over the course of a lifetime," note Rubinstein and Parmelee.[13] For a place to have the significance of home, they write, it must be imbued with a sense of meaning—where important life experiences take place, or where our sense of self is embodied.

In fact, older people can adapt well to change, if the change is tolerable. My mother is a good example. She is not given to spontaneity or adventure, preferring a quiet routine. But at age eighty-four, after recovering from a fall in which she broke both wrists, she decided for herself she wanted to move. She left her home of forty years that she had shared with my father until his death in 1991 and moved into an independent apartment on the campus of a continuing-care retirement community. She now uses a walker and has limited mobility, but she has created a new life with many friends. She feels secure and has never regretted her decision.

As Dr. Fullilove explained in an interview, even those who must move to a nursing home may be relieved to leave home if they cannot safely care for themselves, if they are lonely, or if their poor health has become a burden on loved ones. The question is, she said, "Where do you end up? There are ways to organize nursing homes that are fantastic and are supportive of people's growth and development in old age."

One of the most important lessons she and others draw is that people need to feel connected to others, both within and outside the facility. From their first day at a nursing home, residents need to feel welcomed, even celebrated. They should have opportunities to tell their stories and to feel their voices matter. The life of the nursing home should be "seamlessly integrated with everything that's around them, so they can be nourished at the fountain of the larger society. If they're put off to the side, people are not going to do well," said Dr. Fullilove.

What sounds so painfully obvious amounts to a revolution in long-term care. When Steve Shields set out to change Meadowlark Hills, he and a team of staff leaders gathered regularly to identify everything in the nursing home that one would not find in a home. There were the carts with commercial kitchen trays, the rigid daily schedule displayed on the bulletin board, the nurse's station, the little plastic cups for pills, the curtain dividing the bedroom in two, the beeping call lights, and so on. The process of identifying these nonhome features took six months. "I knew we were there," recalled Steve, "when one of the nurses said, 'There's nothing left.'"

He said that today, "it's what you don't see that is so marked. You don't see people woken up in assembly-line fashion. You don't see people raised in the air and dumped in a tub for bathing. You don't see staff with an attitude of 'We know what's best for you.' You don't see name cards with special diets. You don't see people slumping to the side—they're engaged. You do see residents talking to each other. In fact, the beauty of it you have to absorb by seeing the rhythm of relationships. Our commitment to the individuals means the culture will change over time."

Steve tells the story of a visit to Meadowlark Hills by a foundation executive. He took her on a tour of three households that had been created out of the old nursing home wings.

At the first one, he introduced her to the residents and staff, and they visited for a while. As the two left, she asked Steve, "Where are the really sick people?" He replied, "Well, these are folks who would normally be in a nursing home." But he could tell she wasn't satisfied with the answer.

They proceeded to the second household, and the same thing transpired. This time, she asked, "But where are the *really* sick people?" Steve assured her that the residents she was meeting had very high "acuity levels"—measures of impairment such as incontinence or immobility.

After completing the tour of the third household, they stood talking on the sidewalk outside. His guest said, "But, Steve, where are your slumpers?"

Ah, the slumpers. The group in the wheelchairs, gathered around the nurse's station, that we all envision when we hear the words "nursing home." The club we pray we never have to join.

So, where are the slumpers at Meadowlark Hills? I set out to see for myself.

PART II

Stories from the Front Lines of Change

I didn't come here to die—I came to
contribute something to somebody.
—George Garris, assisted-living
resident, the Mount

Chapter 3

"We'll Fly to Paris"
Honoring Individual Choice

Everyone wants to go home. Perhaps that says too much.
Everyone "wants out."
> —Joyce Horner, *That Time of Year: A Chronicle of Life in a Nursing Home*

We're starting to open our eyes more to change. We're trying
to be more open to what the residents want. The staff is
connecting to residents at a deeper level. If someone wants
an ice cream cone, staff will take people out to get one.
We're at a reawakening. We've institutionalized our residents
just as we are institutionalized. Our residents really worry
about how their choices are impacting us. And we have to
reassure them that it makes our jobs easier because they are
happier.
> —Dee Dolezal, director of nursing, the Village

I began my visit to Manhattan, Kansas, at one of those popular chain restaurants that serve artery-clogging breakfasts and endless cups of weak coffee. Steve Shields sat across from me in the booth. He ordered an enormous platter consisting of a three-egg omelet, ham, home fries, and toast, most of which went untouched as he warmed to his subject.

Steve is one of several unlikely heroes leading the fledgling movement to recreate nursing homes. He is the kind of person that every successful enterprise needs—smart, likable, resourceful, a gifted leader. A tall man with receding, sandy-red hair and a mischievous grin, he manages to temper his righteous indignation over nursing home conditions with a wicked sense of humor.

He leapfrogged into the world of nursing homes straight from his career in offshore oil. It was not an obvious choice. He thrived on the high-risk game of oil exploration. He loved the engineering challenges, the travel to exotic places, the camaraderie. To hear him tell it, he could have happily spent the rest of his days in places like Kuwait and Venezuela, then retired young with enough socked away to loll around on a beach in Mexico.

But in 1991, he was called home to Kansas to deal with a disturbing chain of events. His mother had been diagnosed with Alzheimer's, his father had Parkinson's, and his brother had just learned he had HIV, contracted through a blood transfusion for kidney disease.

Suddenly his priorities were turned upside down. The rush of finding the next big reservoir under the Black Sea paled in importance to finding good care for his family. He went from knowing nothing about nursing homes—"I didn't even know how to spell continuing-care retirement community"—to full immersion in long-term care. He gave up his work, took some courses at Kansas State, and before long was on the fast track in nursing home ad-ministration. He was soon offered the top post at Meadowlark Hills.

Meanwhile, his mother had been moved to a traditional nursing home with a decent reputation. Steve realized that something was dreadfully wrong, though, the day his mother was knocked to the floor by a worker maneuver-ing a buffing machine. His mother's leg was broken. What shocked Steve was not the accident so much as the attitude of the nursing home. The problem, they implied, was not that the employee was careless. The problem was Mrs. Shields herself. She had been dancing in the halls, they said disapprovingly. Anyone dancing in the halls pretty much got what she deserved.

"As soon as it was practical, we went down in the Meadowlark van, and we got her," said Steve. Several months later, his father also moved to Meadowlark.

As his mother's illness progressed, Steve began spending more time in the nursing home wing—the health-care center, as it was then called at Meadow-lark. He realized that he had been avoiding this part of the complex, prefer-ring to spend his time in the administration offices or with independent or assisted-living residents—anywhere but the nursing home. "It wasn't that old age and infirmity repelled me. I can climb right into bed with a dying per-son and soothe them," he said. "But I was avoiding going to the health-care center. It really bothered me. I thought maybe I was in the wrong job."

During the week that his mother was dying, he witnessed daily life in the nursing home as if for the first time. Things he had taken for granted—because they had always been done that way—suddenly seemed glaringly awful.

For example, his mother's roommate was subjected to his mother's suffering. The flimsy curtain dividing the room did little to shield her roommate from what was going on.

And then he noticed how rushed the employees were—although they treated his mother with kindness (she was the boss's mother, after all)—their efforts fragmented by unbending job descriptions. "All these people were coming in and they were doing their 'function,'" said Steve. "You know, their 'function.' A spiller would come, and then a cleaner-upper would come. It felt like that. I remember going out of her room and going up to this enormous nurse's station and I was standing there and I saw it for the first time. I really saw it. I thought, What the hell is this? I looked at this nurse's station and the dim lights and all these people rushing and the beepers going off and people sitting around the nurse's station"—here he enacts a slumper, with eyes closed, jaw drooping, body collapsed sideways—"and I thought, This is a systems problem. My whole background in offshore oil was systems development. And I thought, You stupid idiot."

Meadowlark Hills, which opened in 1980, was founded by a forward-thinking group of local people, representing several area churches, who wanted more retirement options in their community. From its lofty position atop what passes for a hill in Manhattan, Meadowlark had always been thought of as the country club for the older set. In the public mind, well-to-do folks went to Meadowlark Hills, and poor folks went to Wharton Manor on the other side of town. Steve insists this distinction was never accurate. At any rate, under his leadership, the two merged, Wharton Manor was closed, and today more than half the residents in the nursing home are on Medicaid.

Steve delivered me to Willie Novotny, a good-looking, earnest young man. Mentored by Steve, Willie had held many jobs at Meadowlark. He handed me his business card, which identified him as the assisted-living coordinator, but that was already yesterday's title. "I think the current one is chief operating officer," he said. "Steve's greatest accomplishment has been transforming enough of us into leaders in the organization to carry it forward without him holding it up himself. We've all tried to develop charisma and foresight on our own. Together, we can do a pretty good job."

Willie took me on a tour of the campus. The place had the feel of prosperity. Inside the main building, the color scheme was olive, burgundy, and cinnamon, the carpet was plush, and the furniture looked as if it had just been uncrated. Framed paintings by Kansas artists were on the walls.

It soon became obvious, though, that this would not be the standard tour of a nursing home, which usually focuses on amenities such as the dining room, the rehab center, and so on. If residents have any choices in their meals, you will see a menu, along with the weekly calendar of activities. You may or may not be allowed to converse with aides or residents. If the place smells bad, the tour guide will assure you that "it's not usually like this."

But Willie Novotny did not act as if he were trying to sell me real estate. He spoke about the struggle of changing staff members' consciousness and the organizational culture from one that rewards efficiency and institutional convenience to one that honors the choices of individual residents and fosters community. "We don't use terms like 'making the institution better,'" he said. "We want to dismantle the institution and make it home. We view that as sacred. We have a very deep understanding of what we're after."

The next morning, I was invited to have breakfast in one of the households. Steve Shields has banished the words "nursing home" from Meadowlark's lexicon. When I asked him what to call it instead, he said, "I don't know, call it the place where Grandma lives."

Upon entering the building, I saw three front porches, each leading from a common foyer to a household. Each had a different decorating theme, but they all involved rocking chairs, a mailbox, philodendron cascading from hanging pots, and an oak front door framed by curtained windows. The effect was charming and completely unlike the customary nurse's station and gleaming linoleumed line of patient rooms. I rang the doorbell next to a sign that read Ptacek House and waited to be invited in.

A young woman came to the door to greet me. As soon as I entered, I was enveloped by a sense of warmth and tranquility. The living room—upholstered loveseats and armchairs, a television set, and bookshelves with photos of residents and their families—blended into a dining area with wooden café tables that opened to a large country kitchen. There stood a plump, cheerful homemaker—one of Meadowlark's staff positions—cooking at a large stove. She smiled warmly and beckoned me with her spatula to have a seat wherever I wished. The few residents seated at tables eyed me curiously.

Overcoming my shyness, I approached a tall, solid gentleman with a square jaw and thinning hair, eating a bowl of cereal. I asked if I might join him. He hesitated—one of his friends usually sat there. But I assured him I would move when his friend arrived, and he seemed pleased to have me.

I chatted with him about his life. He used to farm, but after he retired, he moved to an apartment. "Then I fell, and no one heard me," he said. "I couldn't reach the call light. The cleaning woman found me, and I ended up here." He missed the farm but seemed content. He was enthusiastic about the food at Meadowlark and appeared disappointed when I turned down the second course offered me: biscuits and sausage gravy. We talked about the war in Iraq. He had fought in World War Two, and he hated to see us go to war again.

Other residents drifted in at their leisure, some in wheelchairs, others using walkers. The homemaker greeted each by name and offered coffee or tea—like a seasoned diner waitress, knowing their preference. The residents were well groomed, calm, and pleasant.

I heard nothing but the sounds of home: the splash of juice being poured, the clink of silverware, conversation, soft laughter. As Steve Shields said, what was perhaps most striking was what was absent: no beepers, no disembodied voices over paging systems, no clatter of carts rumbling through halls. No nurse ensconced behind her station, like the captain on the bridge of a ship. Instead, the nurse, dressed in a flowered smock and white slacks, sat at a wooden rolltop desk in the living room, writing in a chart and stopping frequently to tell residents good morning.

And I realized there were no slumpers. It was pleasant and natural, and it felt good to be there.

The Moral Ecology of a Nursing Home

Scenes like this one at Meadowlark are repeated across the country at homes that have undergone a process to transform their culture. These nursing homes share a fierce commitment to normalcy. In an environment as ordinary and as much like home as possible, they believe, elders remain engaged in life.

"There are natural rhythms to how we live in physical space—universally," explained Rev. Garth Brokaw, administrator of Fairport Baptist Home in Rochester, New York, where I would later journey. "Where do you spend your time at home? Around food, around others in your family. There is natural light, plants. All of a sudden we pluck people out, put them in a dormitory and wonder why they have 'behaviors.' We have to wrap our services around their natural rhythms."

Fundamental to this philosophy is restoring the right of individuals to make basic choices about their daily lives, from when they rise to what they wear, whether they'll have spaghetti or a tuna sandwich for lunch, if they prefer a bath at bedtime or a shower in the morning, or whether they'll spend time sitting in the sun reading a mystery or folding laundry, listening to music, visiting with a preschooler, or taking a nap—depending on their mood, rather than on a predetermined schedule. In theory, nursing home residents have the right, through the Nursing Home Reform Law, to choose how to spend their time. But in reality, their lives are prescribed by a regime not of their choosing.

Individual choice is a foundational value of our culture, and independence the narrative upon which our country was built. We admire the pioneers who strike out on their own, even if it means breaking family ties. Unlike societies where generations of families live together, we expect our children to leave the nest and build their own lives, even if they move thousands of miles away. We look down on adults who still live with their parents as being unhealthily attached. As aging parents, we are often reluctant to impose on our adult children by moving in with them. Most older people prefer being alone to being a burden.

As we age, though, exercising our lifelong freedom becomes more difficult. In a society built around the automobile, for example, getting around on our own can be nearly impossible if our vision fails. If we have physical or mental needs great enough to land us in a nursing home, our options for making independent decisions become drastically reduced. We may feel as if we are the same people. But the world treats us differently, and we slowly succumb. Having to ask for help every time we need to use the bathroom or change our clothes fractures our sense of dignity, privacy, and self-reliance. Or we may be unable to ask because our speech or mental capacities have diminished so greatly. Unfortunately, the institutional mindset of the nursing home serves to exaggerate our limitations rather than minimize them.

As former nursing home aide Tom Gass said in an interview, aides were told to respect patients' privacy. "Meanwhile, we're rooting through their underwear! I don't know when it happens, but somewhere along the line, [residents] realize that no matter what they say, it doesn't make any difference. Their words have no effect. What do you do then? How do you cope with that—if you have enough of your mental faculties, and you realize you have no personal power left?"

In his book, Gass described Harold, a man still "in his right mind" who had considerable physical problems, weakness, and pain. Gass writes with irony that "we know what's good for him" when the man protests he is too tired to do an activity. "We focus on keeping his body intact, but we don't let his protests hold much sway. We count his heartbeats while we ignore what great rivers of sentiment may course through his veins. We monitor and measure all sorts of body parts—the kinds of things that the state inspectors can check easily—but we cannot measure the man. . . . We can make him do whatever we want. He's at our mercy. We see his protests as just another obstacle to his care. We overpower his spirit to treat his colon, his skin, and his blood count."[1]

To be fair, aides just try to do their job as they've been trained—keeping the residents clean and well cared for. But nursing homes and our entire health-care system fail to take into account how it feels from the other side. Laura Gilpin, a nurse and the director of the Planetree Alliance, tells of a focus group she held for hospital patients. One spoke of an abusive nurse who came in every hour throughout the night and shone a flashlight in her face to see if she was breathing. Gilpin said, "That's considered good nursing care. We're taught to check that. But there are other ways. You can quietly listen for breathing. It really hit home—what we think of as good nursing care was thought of as abusive. That's what's wrong with the whole system."

A Veterans Administration nurse shared a similar story. Standard practice at some VA homes, too, is to check residents every two hours throughout the night. One resident, a light sleeper, demanded to be left alone. The nurse, who valued residents' rights, agreed to his request. When higher-ups discovered what she had done, they demanded that staff continue to check the resident every two hours. Backed by the medical director, the nurse advocated for the resident. But to no avail. "They said if he didn't like it, he could go live somewhere else," she said.

In her book on her mother's battle with Alzheimer's disease, Carrie Knowles described a scene from the nursing home. After her mother gained ten pounds, a nurse instructed Knowles and her sister to bring their mother healthier food rather than sweets. "She cannot see the forest for the trees," the author wrote of the nurse. "There is no earthly reason to deny Mom anything, not ice cream, jelly doughnuts, chocolate, or if she asked for it salted peanuts, beer and cigarettes."[2]

A June 14, 2006, Associated Press story told, not surprisingly, of a growing trend of older people fleeing nursing homes to assisted-living or home-health services. "I've been a thinking individual all of my life—it was an atmosphere that was totally foreign to me," said one seventy-eight-year-old man of his nursing home experience.[3]

A considerable amount of research confirms the importance of autonomy and control to our well-being, no matter what our age or how dependent we are. In fact, you could argue that the more dependent you are, the more critical it is to have control over as many decisions as possible. Researchers Johnson and Grant noted two factors that most determine how stressful moving to a nursing home is likely to be: whether the move was anticipated or sudden, and *"the extent to which the individual has control or perceives himself to have control"* (emphasis theirs).[4] The issue of control was particularly critical for people who all their lives had been in charge of their environment, the authors found, while those who had been more passive adjusted somewhat better to moving to a nursing home.

Even more important than personality type, though, was the quality of the environment to which the elder moved. "Those who still had mastery and control over their lives adapted well. If the new environment was seen as threatening, the incidence of depression was higher," Johnson and Grant wrote.[5]

The first months of living in a nursing home are particularly stressful, according to numerous studies. Contributing to new residents' sense of stress were "loss of prized possessions, loss of privacy, medical orientation of 'home,' lack of control of menu or time for eating, confrontation with infirmity of others, uncertainty, and allotment of space and roommate."[6] Why would we expect elders to feel anything other than stress in such a predicament? Wouldn't we?

Other studies on the quality of life of nursing home residents confirm that they want as much autonomy as possible. In fact, they ranked autonomy as more important to their quality of life than they ranked meals and bathing.

For decades, Rosalie Kane of the University of Minnesota has studied quality of life in long-term care. In one study conducted for the Retirement Research Foundation, she explored what residents considered very important in terms of control over everyday life. They ranked at the top "leaving the facility for short times," followed by phone use and mail receipt, choice of roommates, activities, food, care routines, money matters, getting up in the morning, going to bed, and having visitors. Asked how satisfied they were with the amount of choice they had in each of these areas, only 21 to 42 percent said they were "very satisfied." Kane concluded that "the typical nursing home in the United States is the nadir for expression of personal autonomy. Few nursing home residents have control over and choice in the basic conditions of their daily life and care."[7]

In his book on stress, *Why Zebras Don't Get Ulcers*, Robert M. Sapolsky, professor of biology and neurology at Stanford University, briefly discusses the ill effects on nursing home residents when they lose control. "I can imagine few settings that better reveal the nature of psychological stress than a nursing home," he writes. In one classic study he describes, by Judith Rodin and Ellen Langer, a group of residents were made responsible for meal choices, social activities, and choice and care of a houseplant. Compared to a similar group who did not have such choices, these residents initiated more social interactions, described themselves as happier, and, "most remarkable of all, the death rate in the former group was half that of the latter" after eighteen months. Other studies cited by Sapolsky had similar results; one even documented improved immune function in nursing home residents who were given more control over their daily lives.[8]

Eric Haider came to Rodin and Langer's conclusions on his own. I interviewed him at Crestview Nursing Home in Bethany, Missouri, where he was then administrator. Crestview was especially impressive because it was a humble, county-owned facility that had once been the poor farm. Eric demonstrated that he could deliver four-star service to residents even as he relied heavily on the state's low Medicaid reimbursement rates.

Over a lunch of "good old home-cooked food," as one resident described it, of oven-baked fried chicken, stewed green beans, mashed potatoes and gravy, and a bowl of fresh strawberries, Eric told me his story.

He was born in India and, although he has lived in the Midwest since he was six years old, he still speaks with a marked accent from his homeland. He began working in a nursing home in the 1980s. He had married a competent and cheerful local woman, Margie Haider, who was then Crestview's director of nursing. (The Haiders have since moved to Florida and continue their work.) Early in his career, Eric said, he struggled to keep up with changing regulations and higher standards. "There was a growing nursing shortage," he said. "I could not keep up with the competition. I lost all my nurses. At one point I had two nurses—one in a wheelchair and the other one who didn't believe in medication." He laughed and shook his head. "I was struggling."

His next venture was an employment agency that supplied nursing homes with temporary staff. "For the first time I began seeing nursing homes as an outsider," he said. "I started to question why did they do things the way they did."

He recalled going to a nursing home and seeing a woman in a wheelchair, screaming and begging for help. Seven aides walked by her without stopping. He asked each of them why. Four of the seven said they didn't hear the woman. Three said she always behaved that way.

In another instance, a woman was crying. An aide stopped, hugged her, and asked how she could help. When the woman said she was hungry, the aide told her she would have to wait to eat. It wasn't time.

He realized he had operated his nursing home in the same way. "I said, I'm going to fix the way we treat people, burn the regulation book, change the culture, and redo the whole nursing home," he said, adding with some import: "I came back with a big mission—I'm going to go where no one has gone before." He went on to develop an approach he calls "the ideal nursing home—person-centered care."

He and the staff came up with simple ways to elicit from residents specific ideas about how their lives would be pleasant and meaningful. A "Wants and Desires" form documented each resident's individual goals, daily routine, personal care preferences, and favorite food and drink, as well as details about life history and habits. The staff was then challenged to creatively meet these desires.

The approach seemed to be as freeing for staff as it was for residents. "This is the only place I've ever worked where I ask to come in on my day off," one licensed practical nurse told me.

The Dignity of Risk

Should people in nursing homes be so autonomous that they are free to make choices that may harm them? The prevailing view, until recently, has been an emphatic no.

In fact, the goal of eliminating risk dominates the culture and mentality of nursing homes. It's no wonder. Regulators, litigators, and insurance companies have downplayed the quality of life for people who live in nursing homes to focus on clinical care and safety—issues that are important, to be sure, and also easier to quantify, such as the percentage of people who have bedsores, who are incontinent, or who fall. This has led to an unbalanced and unhelpful preoccupation with elders' physical ailments to the exclusion of all else—their happiness, emotional health, spiritual needs, longing for companionship, search for meaning, feelings about death, and many other pressing concerns.

We all want nursing home residents to be safe from injury. But an overly protective attitude aimed at eliminating risk leads to smothering residents with good intentions and stripping them of choice and dignity.

Rev. Garth Brokaw of Fairport Baptist Homes comes across as a mild-mannered sort, with his small moustache and glasses and conservative business suit. But he clearly has a rebellious streak when it comes to rules that don't make sense. He recounts the time an employee had the idea to put out a cookie jar as a friendly gesture. "I can't tell you how much furor that caused with housekeeping, because who was going to clean up all those crumbs?" Garth recalled. "And then infection control got into it. Well, everybody sticking their hands in the cookie jar, you know, and Lord knows where those hands have been. Yeah, well, Lord knows where all my kids' hands have been when they stick them in the cookie jar, too."

Despite the outcry, a cookie jar appeared. "Everybody enjoyed the cookies," he said. "It wasn't such a big issue, because the housekeepers were in there getting cookies, too!"

Neither did the Department of Health complain during the next survey. Garth jokes that maybe the surveyors were too busy munching cookies to cite the nursing home for a deficiency. And the cookie sharing did not increase infections. "What I've tried to say with those kinds of things is, you've got to look at the outcomes. If the outcomes are positive—or if they're neutral—then you don't have an issue. Yes, there's a potential—but there are a lot of potentials in life. That's the way it is."

In addition to worries about poor surveys, fears of litigation prompt nursing homes to enforce petty rules. As Tom Gass writes: "The threat of malpractice is by far more central to our operation than the residents' control over their own lives and property. 'Safety first' means safety from lawsuits."[9]

There is no evidence that nursing homes willing to bear some risk in order to give residents more choice have been the target of more lawsuits as a result. In fact, the happier the residents and their families, the less likely they are to sue, said David Green, longtime administrator of Evergreen. "If you're listening to families, there shouldn't be a problem with lawsuits," he said. "Certainly there wasn't for us."

While I was at Meadowlark Hills, I witnessed a small exchange that demonstrated how one woman had embraced the idea that her mother should be free to take risks, if it meant a life with more dignity and control. I was walking with a staff member, Shari Brown, when we encountered the elderly "Mrs. Smith" covered with bruises. "What happened to you?" Shari asked. "You took up boxing again or something?" Despite her jocular tone, Shari looked concerned as she touched Mrs. Smith gently on the arm.

Mrs. Smith smiled ruefully. Her daughter explained that her mother's chair had malfunctioned. A lever had jammed, and Mrs. Smith had been ejected onto the floor. The team leader on Mrs. Smith's floor wanted her to stop using the chair, which is designed to give people with limited mobility the chance to get up and move by themselves. "You're not going to be able to do that anymore," Mrs. Smith was told. "We would rather come in and help you than pick you up off the floor injured."

But Mrs. Smith and her daughter felt differently. "I think she should still be able to have that level of control," the daughter said.

Shari encouraged them to hold firm, and she brainstormed with them how adjustments to the chair could be made.

Compare that approach with what was considered normal not long ago: restraining people "for their own good." Perhaps no issue upsets nursing home reform advocates more than the practice of tying people to a chair or bed, or chemically restraining them with sedating drugs. But much of the public does not understand why physical restraints are so abhorrent. Nursing home maverick Linda Bump said that she has had trouble convincing some family members that restraints are not to be used. Unlike Mrs. Smith's daughter, who embraced the idea of autonomy for her mother, the wife of one resident was overcome with fear that her husband would fall and injure himself. His dementia had progressed, and his wife wanted him restrained day and night. When the staff told her it was not their policy to use restraints, she complained to the doctor. Even he was unaware that restraints are considered poor practice. "He called and told us, 'You better rethink your policies.'" But Linda stood her ground.

In another instance, she was able to sway a family member who wanted a relative to be restrained by asking him to allow himself to be restrained, to see what it felt like. When the family member agreed, Linda said, "It didn't take very long—maybe an hour. We don't realize how free we are. But when you actually physically tie someone, it doesn't take long for them to think falling might not be such a bad alternative."

Donna Babineau, a nurse and clinical educator for Genesis HealthCare, said she would take it a step further. She believes everyone who works with residents should undergo mandatory sensitivity training that would include being restrained in some manner, even if it's a firm hand on your shoulder when you wanted to get up to go to the bathroom. "Until you experience what a resident experiences, it's foreign," she said.

This in no way is meant to minimize the serious effects of falls. My grandmother never recovered after breaking her hip, and it likely led to her death. My mother's fall in which she broke both wrists required full-time care by me and other family members, and led to her giving up her home.

But restraints are an ill-conceived, humiliating, and dangerous way to prevent falls. Considerable research has shown that in their desperation to get out of restraints, nursing home residents can easily become entangled and strangle on them. Studies show that restraining a person in a chair or bed for long periods of time can result in bedsores, weakness, or pneumonia, not to mention depression and anger.

Even bedrails can be dangerous. Between 1985 and 2006, the U.S. Food and Drug Administration received 691 reports of people, most of whom were "frail, elderly or confused," being "trapped, caught, entangled, or strangled" in bedrails. Of these people, 413 died.[10]

There are far safer and more humane alternatives for preventing falls. An article in *Home Healthcare Nurse* lists twenty-eight alternatives to restraints—from modifying the environment to limiting caffeine and sugar, increasing hydration, and providing physical therapy to increase strength and stamina.[11]

Can nursing homes completely prevent people from falling? Of course not. But, argues Linda Bump, "You acknowledge that dignity outtrumps physical safety and hope that people will, as you work with them, appreciate the quality of life more than the prevention."

Kendal, guided by its Quaker philosophy, has gone more than thirty years without once using a restraint. It has been so successful that the State of Pennsylvania funds a training effort so that Kendal can spread its restraint-free methods to every nursing home in the state. In 1995, according to Beryl Goldman of Kendal, 28.6 percent of homes in Pennsylvania used restraints; that number in 2006 was 4 percent.[12]

"We have had our challenges," said Goldman. "We have had families who want restraint use. We said, 'You came here knowing that is not our position. We'll work through this with you, but using restraints is not an option.'" Goldman said Kendal has not been sued for this policy, although in at least one case, a family member moved a resident. "He moved her out into another nursing home where she spent the rest of her days in restraints. She died in restraints," said Goldman.

I asked Steve Shields how he goes about weighing the right of residents to take risks against the legitimate fear they might get hurt. We were sitting at a round table in his large office in Meadowlark's main building. Regulatory manuals and books on organizational change and leadership development packed the shelves. He had carved out time from his always-swamped schedule to talk about what culture change means to residents and staff. I soon realized that my question about risk taking had struck a nerve. He began slowly.

Risk is inherent to being alive. One of the mistakes we have made in long-term care is to eliminate risk. We are so averse to risk, it's funny. We want to make human file cabinets out of these nursing homes. We don't want anything risky to happen. We're so averse to risk that we'll tie people up to avoid it. We will eliminate life's enjoyment to avert it. And attorneys gobble it up, when risks are taken.

But the fact is, getting up in the morning is a risk, from the moment we're born to the day we die. And in fact every person makes a choice to have two eggs over easy or a hamburger with fries. We're aware that there's risk to our vascular system, and we eat that hamburger. We know that driving has risks. As we get ready to go in the morning, there's a chance that we may not make it to work, or we may not make it back home. But we calculate it, we make a decision, and we drive to work. As a parent with a seven-year-old child, if I really thought about avoiding anything that would keep my child from being injured or from anything happening to his mother or me until he grew up, we would be hermetically sealed in a room.

So we all make choices. Life is full of risk. We make peace with that, we calculate that, sometimes without even really thinking about it. And we build a fabric in our lives. Some of us skydive. Some of us quilt. Some of us take a bus, some take a train, some of us fly, some of us drive a car, some of us don't drive at all. We have made our decisions about where we fit into all that, relative to risk. And there's no acceptable reason that any influence, whether it be regulation or attorneys—nothing should interrupt a person's sense of continuing that dynamic about life.

By now, Steve's voice is rising, and his usually amiable face is clenched in anger. "Shame on us," he said. "Shame on us. That we had to go through decades of tying people to chairs. Shame on us. Where were we? What were we thinking, that we did that? My feeling about risk is, *we take it*. We take it and we facilitate others in negotiating their own."

Oatmeal as a Seditious Act

In the 1986 comic movie *Tough Guys*, Archie Long (Kirk Douglas) and Harry Doyle (Burt Lancaster) are two aging criminals who have spent thirty years in the slammer. Upon their release, Harry's whippersnapper parole officer (Dana Carvey) tells Harry, seventy-four, he must go live in the Golden Sunset Retirement Home. Tyrannical staff control this quasi-assisted-living/nursing home facility. "Too many rules to suit me," Harry grumbles to a friend. When he shoves aside a tray of unpalatable food, a muscle-bound aide tells him in a saccharine voice, "If you don't eat your food, Mr. Doyle, I'm going to be very upset."

"We wouldn't want that to happen now, would we?" asks Harry, heaving the plate of creamed spinach on the aide's white slacks. "Tell the cook me and the boys don't like this crud. We want real food, real food, real food," he shouts, pounding the table with his fist with each declaration. The long tables of elderly men and women delightedly join in, chanting "Real food! Real food!"

Harry Doyles are in short supply in nursing homes, but plenty of residents struggle to exert their will against what seem insurmountable odds. In many cases, as Garth Brokaw observed, these minirebellions are classified as "behaviors." "Behaviors" are nursing home-speak for acting "inappropriately." If a resident resists being bathed, it goes down in her chart as a "behavior." If she dumps her food, à la Harry Doyle, it would certainly be a "behavior." Of course, hauling off and slugging an aide is a terrible "behavior" that happens in nursing homes.

Behaviors are usually attributed to dementia, and the perpetrators are medicated to control their outbursts.

But drugs may not always be the answer to outrageous—or outraged—behavior. Often the institutional culture itself is to blame. By returning to residents as much personal decision making and freedom of movement as possible, some nursing homes demonstrate that many "behaviors" disappear. At Crestview, for example, after person-centered care was initiated, the staff could better anticipate what triggered "behaviors," and the use of drugs went down. From 1998 to 2000, the number of prescriptions for psychotropic medications declined from 27 to 20, anti-anxiety drugs from 40 to 14, and those for sleeping medications from 11 to 2.[13]

Balancing an individual's desires when they run counter to what we feel is in the resident's best interest can be difficult, especially when the resident has

dementia or other mental disorder. At Heritage Manor in Lowell, Massachusetts, Director of Nursing Andy Andreopoulos described a resident who had
formerly been homeless. He escaped (known as "eloped" in nursing homes)
and went back to living on the street. When he was spotted picking food out
of a dumpster, the staff corralled him back. When he refused to shower, they
bribed him with new clothes from the Salvation Army. "You could argue it's
his right to choose to be dirty. He has not yet been deemed incompetent,"
said Andy. "We've got our challenges."

At Pleasant View, in Concord, New Hampshire, I witnessed another small
example of how challenging it can be to solicit input from some residents.
The staff wanted to decorate an alcove where the residents came through a
buffet line. The plan was to cover the green walls with a scenic mural. Barbara Platts-Comeau, the recreation director and culture-change leader, felt it
was important for residents to choose the mural. After all, they were the ones
who would look at it every day at mealtime. At a gathering of a dozen residents, she carefully explained the issue and held up a large wallpaper book.
To make the decision manageable, she had narrowed the choices to three. I
looked around at the group. A young man with severe Down's syndrome was
grunting loudly and trying to grab magazines off a shelf. Another woman hol-
lered at him to stop making that noise. Two people were dozing. Some looked
perplexed. Only a few seemed to be following what Barbara was saying.
Nevertheless, she went around the circle from person to person, patiently
explaining again what she was asking, showing each person the pictures, and
soliciting his or her view, even that of the young man who was not able to express his opinion. In twenty minutes, she managed to get opinions from most
of the group. I felt exhausted just observing the process. But Barbara seemed
energized. After the meeting, she set out down the hall to get more opinions.
"Mr. Jackson," she called cheerfully, "I need you to vote on something." The
man, seated in a wheelchair, slowly lifted his head and smiled kindly at her.
He seemed game for looking at the heavy wallpaper book as she set it on
his lap.

When I described the mural-selection scene to Pleasant View administrator Mark Latham, he smiled. He thought the time well spent. But he
acknowledged the process is counterintuitive. In the past, he said, "I would
have wanted to select the mural myself. It would be done, and we could move
on. We're not particularly good at helping [residents] make these decisions.
It slows things down. I'm rewiring myself to spend more time listening to
what they want."

To encourage people to stay engaged and to voice their opinions, Barbara
solicits ideas at monthly community council meetings open to all residents
and their families. The Nursing Home Reform Law gave residents the right
to have councils, although residents in many nursing homes have not orga-

nized them. When Barbara came to Pleasant View in 2000, the council was barely functioning. Five people came to the first meeting she convened. "Two fell asleep, and the other three were angry," she recalled. "They said, 'We come all the time and no one listens to what we say.'" Barbara was careful to follow through on their first two requests, and gradually she and Mark Latham gained their trust. The meetings grew so large that each floor of Pleasant View has its own council of residents and family members as a way to forge a tighter sense of community.

At lunch I dined with three women and asked them about life at Pleasant View. Although each yearned to return to her own home, they all recognized that the nursing home was trying to accommodate their wishes. One, for example, had requested at a community council meeting that hooks be hung in the bathing room. "I went in the bathroom and saw the hooks, and I said, 'Son of a gun, they did it,'" she told me.

Although resident choice at times may seem more labor intensive for staff, it can save time otherwise spent cajoling recalcitrant residents. Carol Johnson, a geriatric psychologist in Ohio, tells of a consultation she performed several years ago. She was called to a nursing home because a resident became combative every time she had to take a shower. To deal with this unpleasant behavior, the nursing home physician had prescribed Haldol, an antipsychotic drug. But in only a few minutes of conversation, Johnson discovered that the woman simply didn't want to take her shower at 5:30 PM—her assigned time—because that was when her daughter might visit. When the woman's shower was switched to the morning, she no longer resisted and the Haldol was discontinued.

Showers are often difficult for both residents and aides, who bear the brunt of "behaviors." Clinical nurse specialist and Pioneer Network leader Joanne Rader, who specializes in caring for people with dementia, said she got tired of "hearing the screams coming out of the shower room." She decided to figure out a better way to bathe people.

"The staff is not to be blamed," she said. "The system has become so medically oriented or industrially oriented they don't even think it's bad care." To better understand why so many residents get upset about showers, Joanne asked an aide to give her a shower. "It's not a pleasant experience," she said. "Someone takes off your clothes, takes you into a room that looks like a car wash or torture chamber. It doesn't feel very private. It's cold. If you have dementia, it's often painful and scary."

She developed a new approach to bathing using massage and no-rinse soap to clean people while they are still in their beds. "People who would fight like cats and dogs in the shower would act totally blissed out," she said, recalling one formerly obstreperous lady who so enjoyed her bed bath she wanted to give Joanne a tip. Joanne's technique, called "bathing without a battle," has been endorsed by professional nursing organizations and is now in use in many nursing homes around the country.

Contrast this solution with that of a nursing home in Chicago that was featured in a National Public Radio story a few years back. There, as is common, people were lined up in the halls for their turn in the shower room. The aides, who wore white uniforms, found that shower duty was incredibly stressful, often entailing physical tussles, as many of the residents became agitated. It turned out that it was a Jewish nursing home and many of the residents were Holocaust survivors. Imagine how the sight of white-coated attendants forcing them into line for the shower room triggered their deepest fears from the death camps.

So what was the solution? The aides changed to street clothes. Although apparently this did help allay some residents' fears, it seems depressingly short on imagination. Why are people lined up for showers in a public hallway—often with only a sheet draped over them—in the first place? Would *you* want to be bathed that way for the rest of your life?

When Joanne Rader addresses groups, she gives people an assignment. "Go in a nursing home and arrange for people to bathe you." She pauses and allows this suggestion to sink in. "Why is that such a horrible thing to think about? You know what? The reason you don't want to do that is exactly the same for the residents. And yet we label their refusals as aggressive, demented behavior. There is no 'we-they.' It's just a normal response to an uncomfortable situation."

At Crestview a group of staff related how they tried to make bathing a pleasant experience.

Explained one aide, "We had a lady that would not go for her bath. There was a lady in housekeeping who was very close to her. So we would go and get the housekeeper, and she'd go right into the shower room with her." (Allowing a housekeeper to take a break from mopping floors to help comfort a resident in the shower room is not standard procedure in most nursing homes.)

Others in the group chimed in:

"We do bubble baths, we do soft music, we try to decorate the bathroom like their homes."

"We try to keep their bath routine like they did at home. If the resident is able to, they tell us how many times and when they like to bathe—or the family member lets us know. If they had their bath before they went to bed, we try to give it to them then."

"And if they want it every day, they get that—they don't get that twice-a-week routine or whatever they do in other homes."

"We've even given showers at three o'clock in the morning, because that was the resident's preference. It's just whatever they want."

The same attitude extended toward eating. Food choice is basic to our autonomy; we all want to choose what we eat. Ideally, mealtime is a source of sensory pleasure and of camaraderie.

"Most nursing homes, if a resident wakes up and wants to have pizza, they'll say, 'Sorry, we don't have pizza today.' What we say is, 'Okay, do you want to go to Pizza Hut or would you like us to get you carryout?'" said administrator Eric Haider.

Garth Brokaw tells the story of a new resident at Fairport Baptist who wanted to have hot oatmeal every morning. The well-meaning dietitian, schooled in traditional nursing home culture, told him he should have more variety. "This was a man who had lived fine for ninety-two years until now," Garth said. "Had eating oatmeal every day harmed him? Maybe he had lived to ninety-two *because* he had eaten oatmeal every day." The dietitian was reminded that residents could choose whatever they wanted to eat, and the man continued to have his daily oatmeal.

But what if he hadn't been afforded this choice? What if he had then refused to eat? Or what if in frustration he had dumped his poached egg and toast? Would he have been having a "behavior" and put on antipsychotic medication?

At Seattle's Providence Mount Saint Vincent (the Mount), Meadowlark Hills, and other places I visited, aides said that at first, resident choice seemed as if it would take more time and be less efficient. But in the end, the opposite was true. Marsha Wilson, an aide at the Mount, explained the link between staff empowerment and resident choice.

"It's a very nice philosophy compared to other places I've worked, where residents didn't have much choice," she said. "[Residents] tell you what they want. It makes it a lot easier because you don't have the nurses force you to force them to do what they don't want to do. Before, you had to tell them they had to do it, and they did it.

"We get very close because we're able to communicate more. We know residents have rights here. We don't have to run to the nurses if someone doesn't want to do [something]. We just explain why it's beneficial, and if they don't want to do it, that's fine."

Noel Petitjean, former director of nursing at the Mount, recalled how they used to operate, before they set about to change the culture to one they call "resident directed." "At 5:30 AM the aides flipped on the lights in the Alzheimer's unit—then they wondered why people were combative," she said. "When we let people sleep in, we learned we had had them very carefully scheduled for our convenience. We learned that meds and treatments could be at the residents' timing. We were there for their lives, not to make our work handy."

At the Mount, people have six choices about where they eat: their room, their "neighborhood," a sit-down restaurant-style dining room, a cafeteria, an espresso bar in the gift shop, and a morning room with continental breakfast. The cafeteria is bright and sunny, with large-scale images of Seattle. In addition to hot meals, deli food is available all day—as are ice cream, doughnuts, chips, juice, and fruit. What about people who are diabetic? "We encourage them to eat well," said Noel. "But it's their choice. If they were still living at home, they would eat what they want. This is their home. The whole goal is if they want an egg at two o'clock in the morning, you can make it for them."

Why is this concept so foreign to most nursing homes? Noel explained how difficult it is for some nurses to give up control. She herself felt "15 percent offended, 60 percent bewildered, and 25 percent enthused" when she first heard what "resident-directed" meant. "Some RNs [registered nurses] felt very threatened by allowing people to make informed choice about their medical care—refusing meds, eating unhealthy food," she said. "I've interviewed RNs who couldn't work here because a diabetic who wanted ice cream could get it. It's hard for nurses to accept we're not going to change habits of a lifetime."

I have heard similar tales repeatedly. In fact, many transformative nursing homes lost nurses along the road to change.

"I had a nurse who said the problem with this place is residents have too much control," said administrator Mark Latham of Pleasant View. "For generations, we have been task oriented. This is the end result."

In the journal *Home Healthcare Nurse*, Connie Vaughn Roush and Josephine E. Cox discuss this challenge. "Most nurses new to home and hospice care find the level of client control over the care environment difficult and uncomfortable. Often, they have worked in hospitals, places designed and centered around the work of healthcare. Hospital routines and arrangements are predictable and useful to nurses but clients and their families desire an environment that is centered on their individual and family needs. Nurses need to be aware of this need for client control and respect it."[14] Although Roush and Cox are discussing home care, the same could be argued for nursing homes.

Restoring choice to people who are very old and frail may not result in dramatic changes that are obvious to an outsider. "You're not going to see our residents in three-inch heels doing the cha-cha," as Steve Shields puts it. People's wishes may be so modest as to seem inconsequential. But small things matter more as your world narrows.

Steve loves to tell the story of Ida. She was one hundred years old but she had never been a slumper. Before Meadowlark's transformation, Ida had remained engaged by sitting in front of the nurse's station and thinking mean thoughts about every person who passed by. Often she would voice these thoughts, loudly informing a nurse, say, that she could stand to lose about fifty pounds.

As the culture of Meadowlark changed, Steve was eager to show residents how their lives would be different. Ida, he reasoned, would be the perfect person on whom he could test this new approach. He sat down with her and asked, if she were able to spend a whole day doing anything in the world, what it would be. He was prepared to fly to Paris with Ida, he claims, if that was her heart's desire. But Ida couldn't come up with anything she wanted.

He told her he would give her more time to think about it. He returned the next day but to his disappointment she said, "I'm too far gone." She could think of no special way to spend a whole day that didn't seem overwhelming.

Deflated, Steve called LaVrene Norton and told her this whole resident-choice idea wasn't working. He recalled, "LaVrene said, in her nice way, 'You idiot. You overwhelmed the poor woman. You've given her no choice for the last ten years of her life, and now you want to give her a whole day? Go back. Narrow it down to five minutes.'"

This time, he asked Ida, if she could choose what to do for just five minutes, at any time of day, what it would be. She didn't hesitate. She said she would watch the sunrise and drink a cup of her favorite tea in a Staffordshire china cup. That was the kind of china her mother had.

He had to buy a set of eight, Steve said, but it was worth it. From then on, Ida woke at dawn, gazing out the large windows at the field surrounding Meadowlark and sipping Earl Grey in a Staffordshire china teacup. Such a simple daily ritual, but one she had not been able to enjoy since moving to the nursing home.

"How much have we been taking away from people, in our blindness?" Steve asked.

Chapter 4

"We Are Nothing"
Empowering Staff

All the affection, all the consoling, all the filling of emotional
holes and the tidying up of frayed feelings are invisible to
the owners, to the administration, and to the official state
regulators who monitor us so closely. . . . I have never known
of any aide being rewarded or recognized for being kind.
— Tom Gass, *Nobody's Home: Candid Reflections of a
Nursing Home Aide*

We know our residents. We know their wants and needs.
We know pretty much what's going on. We set up our own
budget for activities. It's not a control thing anymore. You can
make decisions, and it's all about what the residents want.
— Sherry Smith, aide at Meadowlark Hills

In the conference room at Crestview Nursing Home in Bethany, Missouri,
a dozen or so staff members were given time out of their workday to talk
with me about their jobs. Crestview had a far different feel from Meadowlark
Hills. Originally the poor farm, Crestview remained a low-budget operation
owned by the county. The conference room where we sat still had the track
on the ceiling, demarcating where curtains once offered scant privacy in a
four-person ward.

But Crestview had risen from its once lowly state. At the time I visited, it
was viewed as a national model for long-term care. One advocate described
it as the "most liberating" nursing home she had ever visited.

I asked the staff what made Crestview different from other nursing
homes.

"It's not as institutionalized as the others," said Cissy, a young aide whose mane of curly red hair was pulled back in a ponytail. "You get to have fun with the residents. You don't get in trouble for sitting down and talking to a resident."

A licensed practical nurse spoke up, saying she drove forty miles a day to work there, even though several other nursing homes were closer to her home. She had tried working at one of them. "That was a job," she said. "This is family. The other places didn't follow our standards."

I asked them how they learned their approach to working at Crestview. At first, they thought I meant the basic training they received to do their job. Crestview, like other nursing homes, required aides to successfully complete a seventy-five-hour classroom course and a hundred hours on the floor to become certified. Aides were taught how to bathe, feed, and transfer (help move) residents. They learned to observe symptoms to see if residents were in pain or losing range of motion. They took residents on walks and collected urine specimens. "You learn all that," said Charlie, an aide and staffing coordinator. "But then we add the fun to it."

This was the second time the word "fun" had come up, and I pointed out that "fun" is not a word that most people associate with nursing homes. In fact, I said, in many nursing homes I've heard people moaning or calling for help.

"They're scared. They want to make sure there's someone there besides them," Cissy explained. "So that means staff is not really interacting with them, so they think they're the only person there. And if you don't go in that room once in a while, they get scared. We're in the room all the time."

"You're not sitting around the nurse's station," I observed.

They all burst out laughing. "You better not!" someone called out.

"We're here for them," said Charlie. "It makes them feel needed and wanted."

"What we have is one big family," said Tammy, the social worker. "These residents are more like our grandparents. Residents ask about the employees. When I had my baby, I got calls and cards. One lady even came to the hospital. They become a part of our lives. They ask about our kids."

Carla, another team leader, regretted the years she spent working in a factory, even though she earned more on the assembly line than she does at Crestview. "These residents give me far more than we give them," she said. "It makes all your problems seem small. They make me feel very, very special. That's worth more than high wages."

The joy and confidence these staff members expressed is all too rare in nursing homes. Staff turnover and a shortage of direct caregivers have created a crisis in long-term care. Annual turnover among aides in nursing homes is 70 percent nationally; in ten states it is over 100 percent. Turnover among nurses, including directors of nursing, is nearly 50 percent. Vacancy rates are high. Some 52,000 aide positions go unfilled in nursing homes, while 14,000 registered nurses and 25,000 licensed practical nurses are needed. According to state ombudsmen data, from 1996 to 2000, complaints from families and residents about staff turnover rose by 208 percent.[1]

The pioneers who set out to radically reform nursing homes recognized early on that the institutional culture was as detrimental to the health and well-being of staff as to that of residents. Successfully tackling this critical problem is a hallmark of transformative nursing homes. In places such as the Mount and Traceway's Green Houses in Tupelo, Mississippi, for example, staff turnover has plummeted to 15 percent and 10 percent respectively. Transformative homes are learning that the more respect and responsibility aides are given and the more time they can devote to relationships with elders, the happier both aides and elders are.

Who Cares for our Elders?

- Numerous job openings and excellent job opportunities are expected.
- Most jobs are in nursing and residential care facilities, hospitals, and home health care services.
- Modest entry requirements, low pay, high physical and emotional demands, and lack of advancement opportunities characterize this occupation.

> —U.S. Bureau of Labor Statistics, *Occupational Outlook Handbook, 2006-2007*, on Nursing Aides

The typical aide in a nursing home is a woman (90 percent); the average age is thirty-seven. Half have a high school diploma or GED, and 27 percent have at least some college. Nearly half are women of color, often immigrants whose English skills may be poor. Their median hourly earnings in 2004 were $9.86, although some earn as little as $7.00 or as much as $12.00. One-fifth earn incomes below the poverty level, and one-fourth to one-third are the sole support of their families.[2]

Among nursing home staffers, these "direct care" or "front-line" workers have the most contact with residents. Studies estimate that aides provide 80 to 90 percent of care.

The lives of aides and residents are interconnected in strong and complex ways. Their relationship represents the potential either for true intimacy, friendship, and mutual support or for cruelty and indifference. Most people who choose to work in a nursing home start out feeling a basic concern and sympathy for older people. But whether these good instincts flourish or burn out depends more on the environment in which aides work than on individual character.

If you live in a nursing home, an aide will wake you up in the morning, help you to the bathroom or onto the bedpan, clean you up if you have soiled yourself, assist you in dressing, make sure you get to the dining room, help you eat if you need it, walk you through the halls, and so on. The first face you see in the morning and the last you see at night will be that of an aide. Your well-being, your very life, is in her hands. If she doesn't give you good skin care, you develop a bedsore. If she doesn't take the time to help you eat properly, you will become malnourished or you may aspirate and succumb to pneumonia. If she fails to fill your water pitcher—and to leave it within reach—you will become dehydrated. If she doesn't respond to your call light when you have to go to the bathroom and you try to get there yourself, you are at risk of falling and breaking a hip. You are at her mercy.

Often complicating this relationship are cultural, economic, and language differences between the lowest-paid workers in a nursing home on one hand—the nurse's aides, kitchen aides, housekeeping staff—and the nurses, administrative staff, and many residents on the other. This is true not only in the United States, but also increasingly around the world. A study by AARP found that "the most intimate care to frail older persons in developed countries is increasingly provided by young women whose native language, race, and culture are different from those they serve."[3]

Former aide Tom Gass described himself and his coworkers as "society's castaways. . . . Typically aides give their lives away to strangers, while they themselves drive old cars and suffer bad teeth." He adds that, while the field draws a small share of petty thieves and sex offenders, "most aides are good and decent people who would love nothing more than to work their way up into the lower middle class."[4]

A study conducted in Kansas on improving staff communication in nursing homes uncovered among aides "a sense of cynicism with one's fellow human beings among study participants. These feelings are characteristic of people who have experienced a great many hard times and disappointments."[5]

To this often beleaguered group we entrust the most vulnerable members of society, our frail elders. The work is backbreaking and often messy. Aides deal with a duty that most of us would find incredibly difficult: keeping people clean who are incontinent—or people who have become incontinent because no one has regularly assisted them to the bathroom in a timely manner. Psychiatrist Lori L. Jervis has discussed the symbolism of "pollution" and "dirty work," and the effect of such work on aides' self-esteem. Aides hone strategies, including bravado, humor, and finding meaning in sacrifice for others, to handle this difficult task and to deal with the attitudes of disgust from outsiders, she writes.[6]

One aide told me that her coworkers often thought of themselves as mere "butt wipers." Another aide spoke of the challenges of working with people with dementia, including a man who made balls of his feces and threw them at the aide. "What do you do when that happens?" I asked in horror.

"Duck!" he said, laughing.

While reports of cruelty against nursing home residents are widespread, far fewer have considered the problem of cruelty against aides. Aides routinely face physical assault from people with dementia. And it's not only residents who abuse aides. A survey of seventy long-term care administrators found that family members also verbally and physically assaulted staff. Over a six-month period, these administrators reported nearly twelve hundred verbally aggressive acts and thirteen physically aggressive acts against staff. The U.S. Bureau of Labor Statistics found that aides working in long-term care represent the occupation *most at risk* of workplace assault. In a study of a violence-prevention program, focus groups of aides from six nursing homes, three rural and three urban, described routine incidents of violence with which they were confronted, including "hitting with a hand or object, scratching, pinching, biting, grabbing, pulling hair, twisting wrists, poking, spitting, and throwing objects," not to mention verbal assaults that included threats, cursing, racial slurs, and other insults. Every aide in attendance had experienced violence. It is worth noting that of the six nursing homes in this study, one had far fewer problems. In this home, aides received considerably more respect from supervisors, and the leadership was team based rather than hierarchical, with everyone helping out at mealtime, no matter their job title. Whether or not this home described its staffing pattern as "culture change," that is in fact what was going on.[7]

In addition to assaults, nursing home staff routinely face on-the-job injury, and back problems in particular. According to a study by the Service Employees International Union, working in a nursing home is more dangerous than working in a coal mine, a steel mill, or a construction site.[8]

Working Short

As maddening as it is for residents to be woken up early each day to eat a breakfast not of their choosing, it can be just as disheartening for the aides who must disturb their sleep. If you are an aide, your day might well have begun hours earlier, getting your own children up against their wishes. Many aides do not earn enough to own a car and must rely on public transportation. Regardless, you must punch the time clock in time to be on the floor, ready to work, by 7:00 AM. Being late is bad; your coworkers on the night shift are ready to go, many to pick up their own children before heading either home to collapse or perhaps to a second day job. Too many tardies, and you may get docked a day's pay. You get your assignment for today: fifteen residents to care for, instead of the usual ten. Too many aides are out today, so you'll be "working short." And not only are you working short—again—but the residents you have are especially difficult. Mr. Hamm, for instance, is obese, and your back already is aching. Another has extreme dementia and has struck out at aides or pulled their hair.

You get right to work. As at many nursing homes, the residents have already been rousted by the night shift and are waiting to be taken to breakfast. Some need your immediate attention to begin their morning routine. The obese man has been left for you to get up. You try to find help to lift him. A call light dings down the hall, signaling that another resident needs you. But you have already told Mr. Hamm that you will be right with him, so you ignore the light. You finally convince someone to help you. By the time you have Mr. Hamm situated, three more call lights have come on. The woman with dementia is yelling at ear-splitting volume, "Marge, why did you leave?" over and over again. Who is Marge? No one knows, but this resident always calls for her in great anguish. You are aware of the charge nurse looking at your call lights and wondering why you aren't more on the ball. She doesn't offer to help you.

Meanwhile, most of your residents are still sitting there, hoping to get to breakfast before the scrambled eggs are cold.

"I went home crying every night because of what I couldn't get done," one aide told me of her first job in a nursing home "Everything was done assembly-line fashion. It was horrific. No one cared."

The notion of health care as assembly-line work is not unique to nursing homes. As a dialysis technician, I faced similar pressure. A supervisor once chastised me for spending a few minutes talking with patients as I put them on the dialysis machine, a painful, stressful experience that involved having large needles stuck into their arms. "You're holding up production," he told me, without irony.

For years after, I had a recurring nightmare: I arrive at the dialysis clinic, which has expanded, in the way of dreams, to the size of a basketball stadium, filled with patients. I am the only one who has showed up for work that day, and all eyes are on me. I desperately set to work. At the machine of the first patient, I find that half the supplies are missing. I go to find a clamp, and when I return, I realize I need gloves, and so on. In the nightmare, I never get even one patient started on treatment, and the others all wait, staring, like an accusing jury. I feel panicky and helpless. My intentions are the best, but the whole game is rigged for me to fail.

The tales of aides in far too many homes across the country mirror those nightmare feelings. "I used to be accused of spoiling the residents. I was told, don't talk to people, don't give a graham cracker to someone who's hungry," a nurse said of her early experience as an aide.

Caregiving as medicalized assembly-line work is described at length by Timothy Diamond in *Making Gray Gold: Narratives of Nursing Home Care.* Diamond was a university researcher who worked for years as an aide in several nursing homes to gain an understanding of the work. From inside the belly of what he called the "medical-industrial complex," he described the frenetic pace. One head nurse instructed aides to confine all residents in the dayroom, tied to chairs in vest restraints, following their "feedings." "Sometimes there will be only three of you instead of four on duty when we're short on another floor," she told them. "We like to know where they are at all times. So keep them in here after meals. It's more efficient."[9]

Diamond continued: "'Efficiency' was a favorite word, as it is in all businesses, and in these settings, as elsewhere, it was tied to the labor force and the abilities of the administration to produce the product with the fewest employees, within a specific calculus of labor costs . . . Upstairs as the day went along we coped with demands far exceeding our capacities—'Wait for me, will you?' 'Water, please give me some water,' 'Are we going to the funeral now?' 'Stay with me'—a constant stream of requests cascading down the hallways amid the clamor of the call buttons."[10]

Diamond even described a speedup much like those driven by time-study experts on any factory floor. In this case, aides were summoned to the administrator's office to be scolded for not working fast enough. The administrator then announced a plan to make their day even more task oriented (rather than person oriented), designed for top "efficiency." Instead of four aides on a floor for every sixty or so patients, they would work with three-and-a-half: one to do all the toileting, one to do the showers and beds, one to be in the dayroom with the residents, and the "half" to float between floors.[11]

To be fair, Diamond's experience took place when restraint use was common, before the passage of the Nursing Home Reform Law. But study after study of staff turnover in nursing homes today echoes his concerns about efficiency and overwork. A report by the Nursing Home Community Coalition of New York State revealed a depressing litany by aides: "So much responsibility. I feel so guilty because I can't do what I should do." "We are seen only as feces cleaners." "We want to be part of the community." "I can't get supplies—diapers, towels, soap—to do my work." "I can't give enough care. I am always rushing. I feel so bad that my blood pressure is going up. I can't take it." "We are nothing."[12]

In the Kansas study mentioned earlier, which aimed at improving communication between aides and nurse supervisors, participants reported that they worked short more than 70 percent of the time, with staff having to race from one thing to the next without ever catching up. "During these stressful times, nurses and aides routinely clashed, aides clashed with other aides, aides felt ignored and badly treated and nurses felt overwhelmed. Stress of this magnitude makes it exceedingly difficult to implement new behaviors," the study noted.[13]

Directors of nursing (DONs) too report growing dissatisfaction with their jobs. A 2006 survey by Novartis Pharmaceuticals found that the top source of frustration for DONs was staff recruitment and retention.[14]

Working short is at least as bad for residents as for staff. At a faith-based facility I visited in Ohio, residents slumped in wheelchairs filled the hallways. The environment was deadly. I asked the charge nurse what she thought of life there generally. "Oh, it's very good," she said. "We're the best around." Perhaps they were. But I wanted to flee. I had already learned from a frustrated relative that her father had not been incontinent when he moved there but had automatically been put in "diapers" because of short staffing and was essentially forced into incontinency because no one had helped him to the bathroom.

According to a study conducted for the Aspen Institute: "Health care researchers have long noted the connection between the quality of direct-care jobs and the quality of care received by clients." Inadequate levels of staffing are associated with increased risk of falls, pressure sores, incontinence, malnourishment, and dehydration. The single most important criterion for measuring the quality of a nursing home is its level of staffing, many experts believe. Yet most nursing homes in our nation—54 percent, according to one study—don't provide enough staff to prevent harm to residents, while 97 percent do not have enough staff to provide all the care required to avoid risk.[15]

Numerous studies establish the link between a stable workforce, adequate staffing, and high quality of care. A 1996 Institute of Medicine report cited research showing that with better staff ratios, nursing homes tended to use fewer restraints and medications, and residents had higher functional improvements and better survival rates.[16]

Working short, already endemic in nursing homes, will probably become even more common. There are simply not enough people willing to take jobs that are so stressful, pay so little, and are so little respected. At the same time, the demand for aides' services will increase substantially, even as the pool is shrinking. The worker shortage has grown so acute that it has actually become *in*efficient; recruitment has become a Sisyphean task for nursing home operators, as a worker disappears out the back door for every new one who comes in the front. A conservative estimate of what it costs a nursing home to replace a single aide is $2,500 in advertising, recruitment, and training. Annually, staff turnover costs the average home $150,000, while absenteeism adds an additional $75,000 burden. Nationally, the cost of turnover among frontline caregivers is estimated at $4.1 billion annually, $2.5 billion of it borne by the taxpayer through Medicare and Medicaid.[17] This includes costs for advertising, drug screening and preemployment physicals, staff time to interview and check references, orientation, and temporary coverage while the position is vacant. In an "industry" that constantly complains of barely making ends meet, this represents a huge drain on tight resources.

A Difficult Job Made More Difficult

Piling on to aides' woes is a hierarchical management structure. Working short might be more bearable if the entire staff pulled together. But instead, traditional nursing homes have a strict hierarchy that often deprives aides of self-respect. The feeling of being disrespected and undervalued—even more than the low wages and difficult working conditions—is at the heart of staff turnover, according to numerous surveys.

Nancy Foner's disturbing ethnography *The Caregiving Dilemma: Work in an American Nursing Home* reports her observation of daily life in a nonprofit nursing home in New York City over the course of eight months in 1988–89. "Aides cannot take a patient off the floor or alter care plans, even adding chair padding, without a nurse's okay," she writes.

> Patient requests often have to go through the coordinating nurse. Should a patient want to stay in bed, the coordinating nurse must grant permission. If a patient asks an aide for a certain kind of food, she cannot call the kitchen herself but must go through the coordinating nurse. . . . Because the coordinating nurses decide work schedules, aides have to go to them with requests for days off.
>
> Some aides had been working in the same rooms, and with many of the same patients, for years and felt proprietary over "their" section. By rotating aides among sections on a floor every few months, the director of nursing aimed to break them of the notion that they owned their sections and to make them easier to supervise.[18]

The result was grim for residents, Foner reports: "At every level of the nursing department, efficiency and organization were valued over compassion to residents." An aide Foner describes as "Gestapo-like" in her bullying and berating of residents was rewarded and praised for her efficient work methods, while a kindhearted aide who lovingly tended residents was chastised for working too slowly.

What makes Foner's book especially troubling is that, unlike Timothy Diamond, she was not working undercover. She was given full access by a supportive administration, which apparently saw nothing about the institution to hide. This is simply the way it was in 1989—and continues to be in far too many nursing homes.

Despite a growing body of research that shows the benefits of giving staff consistent assignments, 90 percent of nursing homes rotate assignments, according to experts writing for the U.S. Centers for Medicare and Medicaid Services.[19] Stated reasons range from wanting to make sure no one gets stuck with the most difficult residents, to protecting staff from grieving when residents die by not allowing them to get too close, to making sure all staff are familiar with all residents, as they may be frequently pulled from one floor to another. (As we will see, no research supports any of these reasons.)

In one study of turnover, conducted through in-depth interviews of aides, University of Wisconsin nursing researcher Barbara Bowers and her colleagues explored how aides (commonly called CNAs or Certified Nursing Assistants) interpret short staffing and low wages. "The CNAs believed facility managers and supervisors treated them individually as if they were all unskilled, dishonest, lazy, and stupid," the authors noted. They learned that the feeling of being disrespected is at the root of dissatisfaction and that many strategies used by administrators to deal with working short only exacerbated aides' resentments. For example, managers frequently turn to temporary employment agencies to contract for extra help. In the managers' view, they were increasing staff-resident ratios and providing extra sets of hands to help aides do the work. But the hiring of temporary workers made aides feel as if managers thought "just anyone off the street" would do.[20]

Supervisors' actions belied their claim to value resident-centered care, aides felt. Hiring temporary workers and pulling full-time aides from floor to floor meant staff could not form relationships with the residents and thus could not provide the best care. The authors noted that aides rightly believed that quality caregiving was based "on the establishment and maintenance of good relationships with residents."[21]

These aides resented even something as simple and well intentioned as an across-the-board wage increase. Why? Because by rewarding slackers and exemplary workers alike, the raise failed to recognize those who went the extra mile for residents. Their resentment does not suggest that aides do not want and deserve more money, but rather shows how important it is to them to be able to do a good job of caregiving and to have their efforts recognized.

"Conventional nursing homes struggle to manage the problem of staff turnover by offering recruitment and retention incentives to *individual* employees," says Bill Thomas. "Those engaged in the work of culture change seek to create a *culture* of faith, trust, honor, and dignity. Experience shows that this approach is far more effective and less expensive than conventional human-resource practices."

In her research, Bowers found that the aides' knowledge and that of nurse supervisors came from different sources; it was almost as if they lacked a shared language of care. Many aides operated with what Diamond referred to as "mother's wit," deep wells of caregiving instinct, so that holding a hand or placing a moist cloth on a brow were valid, effective treatments for pain or discomfort. Nurses, on the other hand, were trained to use treatments that had been clinically tested. They tended to dismiss the old-school ways and intimate knowledge of a particular resident that the aides carried in their heads and hearts.

Working Conditions Most Important to Aides

Having enough staff to care for residents
Being treated with respect
Having the tools to do the job
Being trusted by supervisors and nurses
Having a friendly, trusting relationship with residents and
    families
Having all staff work together as a team
Having a good working relationship with the supervisors and
    licensed nurses
Being informed of any changes before the change
> —From Nursing Home Community Coalition of New
> York State, "What Makes for a Good Working Condition
> for Nursing Home Staff: What Do Direct Care Workers
> Have to Say?" June 2003

Researcher Robyn Stone, director of the Institute for the Future of Aging Services, is a national expert on nursing home quality and staffing. She has learned that while higher wages are important to worker satisfaction and retention, even more important are the personal relationships among staff, management, and residents. One study she cites found that "homes in which nurse supervisors accepted nursing assistants' advice or simply discussed care plans with the aides reported turnover rates that were one-third lower than those without these practices."[22]

She stresses that changing the supervisory structure from top-down to participatory is fundamental to improving conditions in nursing homes. "In so many studies, over and over and over again, the main issue that comes up in the nursing home setting for retention and job satisfaction is the supervisor," she told me. "That's where you are going to get the biggest bang for your buck."

Without a participatory supervisory structure, the rest—giving residents more choices in menus and decorating, making homier environments—will not fundamentally change the culture of nursing homes. This was brought home to me by residents of a for-profit nursing home that was making a serious effort to change its culture. Several residents said they appreciated the changes the administration was trying to make. They felt lucky to be there and believed theirs was the nicest nursing home in the area. One appreciated being able to bring her own belongings, including a bureau she had refinished herself. But they also felt the burden of staff working short. "They're trying to do a lot of things to make it better for us, but what we really need is someone to help us," said one woman, who told me she had recently waited for an hour for someone to answer a call light when she had to go to the bathroom.

A study by Susan Eaton of Harvard University of workforce organization in twenty nursing homes in California and Pennsylvania explores the relationship between worker and resident satisfaction. Eaton identifies three distinct types of nursing homes. Nearly 70 percent reflect what she calls "traditional low service quality," with a rigid hierarchy, low wages, high staff turnover, and a philosophy of care that is "medical-custodial." Twenty percent reflect "high service quality"; these allow input from aides, pay better wages, and have lower staff turnover and a philosophy of care that was "medical-rehabilitative." They are clean, provide good care, and have higher resident activity levels and better social engagement among residents, visitors, and aides.

The remaining few are nursing homes that have undergone culture change. Eaton calls them "regenerative communities," where residents and staff alike are treated as respected, contributing members. According to Eaton: "The results are striking. The most important change was reversing the assumption of [resident] decline, and substituting a paradigm that emphasized dignity, choices, and growth for residents and employees."[23]

The new model, Eaton's "regenerative community," is based on empowerment and teamwork, and it is perhaps the most difficult change of all. Pam Elrod, senior vice president for operations for Genesis HealthCare, describes it as "the art of inclusion"—bringing decisions as close to those they affect as possible. "It's a huge paradigm shift. It's easy to understand superficially, and it's very hard to internalize it in how we behave every day. Whether you're mom and pop or corporate, inclusion has never been the way we've managed. It's always been an inverted pyramid, where the top makes all the decisions. I tell them to invert the pyramid. That's a difficult concept."

Sarah Greene Burger, a nurse herself and a long-timer leader of the nursing home reform movement, explained why inverting the pyramid is difficult for many nurses. "It takes a nurse who is willing to think differently, and boy, it's tough for us," she said. "It's so hard to say, 'Okay the way I've given care for the last thirty years is sorely lacking.' How do you say that to yourself? They have to realize that happens in every profession. As things change, you change too, and that's good, that's how you make progress. You can't look back—you have to celebrate looking forward."

Most staff want to do a good job for the residents in their care. Given this, one research team concluded: "It is time for leadership to become creative and build on that base, providing CNAs with job mobility, job enrichment opportunities, recognition, and increased job responsibility, producing positive outcomes not only for the CNA but also for the resident and the facility."[24]

Eliciting the Best

At a Holiday Inn conference room in Manchester, New Hampshire, workforce consultant Sue Misiorski stood before two dozen managers of Genesis HealthCare and said slowly and deliberately: "Workers don't leave their jobs. They leave their supervisors. If an employee thinks you don't believe in them, they *will* leave you."

Sue, a culture-change expert with the nonprofit Paraprofessional Healthcare Institute, was there to overturn the status quo. Her organization's mission is to help long-term care facilities create high-quality jobs for direct-care workers, with the end goal of providing high-quality care to elders. Through a method called "coaching supervision," Sue and her colleagues train top managers to rethink what it means to lead. They in turn will share what they learned with supervisors within nursing homes in their company.

A nurse supervisor herself before becoming a consultant, Sue told the group that she knew nothing about supervising when she was first put in charge. Nurses are promoted not because of their leadership skills but because of their strong clinical skills—in other words, they are good nurses, but not necessarily good leaders. When Sue was promoted, her company taught her three things that were intended to make her a good supervisor: how to write people up for disciplinary action, how to be in compliance with regulations, and how to keep a union out. People around the room nodded in recognition.

"Just as culture change means person-centered on behalf of the residents," Sue told the group, "coaching is person-centered on behalf of employees."

Through role-playing, games, and exercises in communicating, Sue and her colleagues demonstrated how to build strong relationships between supervisors and aides. In one skit, a supervisor chastised an aide for bad-mouthing permanent assignments. The aide was warned that if she continued to have a bad attitude, she would be written up. The aide was sullen and said little.

Replaying the scene using the coaching method, the supervisor solicited the aide's views, rather than just telling her she was wrong, and discovered the aide had worked at another nursing home where permanent staffing had been a disaster for her. The reason: the aide had been stuck with some of the most difficult residents. The supervisor asked how making consistent assignments could be done fairly. By the end of the conversation, the aide had suggested that she and the other aides should choose for themselves who would care for which residents.

"The role of the coach is to help the direct-care worker to develop their own problem-solving skills, instead of telling them what to do about a problem," Sue later explained.

It's just a wonderful, much more supportive way of being engaged with workers. I find that in health care the supervisory structures that have traditionally been in place are punitive. They make people feel blamed, and it creates a "gotcha" culture. The supervisors talk to you mostly when you've done something wrong. The procedures are quite standard throughout the industry: If you have done something wrong, first you get a verbal reprimand, second a written, then a suspension, and then termination. But there's no support system to help them resolve what they got written up for. So it's completely ineffective. They feel unsupported, blamed, they are treated unfairly, less valued and less respected. When you implement the coaching, it really transforms the relationship between the worker and the supervisor. That's one thing we're doing that is significantly helpful. No matter how good the relationship with the resident is, if the relationship with your coworkers or supervisor is not good, the relationship with the resident is not enough to sustain you.

There are many paths to staff empowerment, but all lead to a single goal: trusting that aides know residents best and thus must be key decision makers in any nursing home. Staff empowerment also means giving aides authority to organize their schedules and workload, and including their opinions in hiring decisions. At Heritage Manor in Lowell, for example, no aide is hired without the approval of the aides who will directly work with her. At many homes, aides now do self-scheduling. A household team plans the schedule to ensure adequate coverage, while honoring as often as possible individual requests for days off. This contrasts with the traditional model, where charge nurses make up the schedule with little input from aides.

Some nursing home managers point out that staff empowerment, while it sounds good in theory, can be difficult to implement, especially for the growing number of immigrants who now work in the caregiving field. "It's scary to be empowered, especially if you have not been empowered before," said Mary Savoy, director of health services at the Methodist Home in Washington, D.C., which is implementing a model called Wellspring. For some immigrants, she said: "This whole notion of empowerment is really something they just cannot adjust to or identify with. I have staff who, when I walk in the room, they stand up and bow. I'm in the front lobby, and they bend over and say, 'Good evening, boss'! It's cultural. That whole notion of empowerment is not as easy as it sounds and not as rewarding to all employees."

On the other hand, she added: "We have several staff who seem to be a natural for this and appreciate the whole notion of empowerment. We have to watch the ripple effect and see how it goes." The staff I interviewed at transformative homes seemed more comfortable, happy, and confident the more responsibility they were given. This directly translates into better care and a higher quality of life for people who live there.

Diane Sinclair, a young aide at Ridgewood Center in Bedford, New Hampshire, explained how her nursing home implemented consistent assignments, a fundamental piece of any culture change in nursing homes. The aides assigned residents to one of five categories, depending on the level of care they needed. They then took turns choosing the residents they wanted, making sure that the care load was equal. "I liked the consistent assignments from the start," she said. "One gentleman on this floor, no one wanted. But now that one person has him, he's not a major pain in the neck anymore." The aide knows him well, so she can anticipate his needs before he becomes belligerent.

Although Diane had ten residents, some needed less assistance than others, and she felt she was able to do her job well. "My routine is down pat," she said. Having consistent assignments is "easier for you and for them." She took obvious pride in her ability to help residents in ways that made her workday easier and their lives more dignified. For example, "I have in my head when they need to be toileted," she said. "One woman who used to be incontinent has been continent now for three months. Their families are really appreciative too. This year I got four cards [at Christmas]. They say things like, 'You ease my mind.'"

Bonnie Kisielewski, administrator of Ridgewood, is proud that she has gone eight years without using agency workers. She believes consistent assignments are a big draw for staff, and one reason they stay.

Marsha Wilson, an aide at the Mount, reflected on her work. "We make a decent wage. Here, they let you know you're appreciated. We have plenty of staff. You can get in trouble for not answering lights. There's a lot of places where [they let residents] sit in a Depends [disposable briefs] all day rather than take them to a bathroom. It's bad. You get skin breakdown, and they get cranky. I always treat these people like I'd want my family treated. The happier you make them, the less they demand of you. I take care of all their needs and joke around with them. They say they hate to bother me. I have patients say, 'You're a gift from God. You're an angel.'"

Many studies on the benefits of consistent assignments support Diane and Marsha's experiences. Not only do staff find the work more satisfying, but residents also reap real health benefits, including a 75 percent reduction in bedsores after one year of consistent assignments, an 18 percent decrease in patient death rate, and a 36 percent increase over two years in the number of patients who could walk.[25]

Hand-in-hand with empowerment of aides go a sense of teamwork and an end to hierarchical management. At Evergreen in Oshkosh, long-time administrator David Green used the innovative "total quality management" business model to transform the culture of the nursing home. As part of this approach, Evergreen created a quality council that included five representatives from the resident-care side—aides, nurses, housekeepers, and activities—and five from administration, including Green as CEO. "With the quality council, we did some things really right," he said. "Everybody had the same vote and decision making. That was radical in and of itself. Staff would go out and say, 'We voted David down again!' The team meant something."

At the Mount, the blending of jobs means that anyone answers a call light, not only the aides. Brenda Jennings, a nurse and neighborhood coordinator who began work there as an aide, jokingly calls herself "the highest paid scullery maid in Western Washington" because she pitches in wherever she is needed. But she's not alone. "The housekeepers will answer call lights. The recreation therapists are trained as CNAs, as are the social workers. Everyone in the building has a food handler's permit, to help out with meals."

Brenda explains why culture change is rewarding not only to aides but to nurses. "RNs have to give up control, but not authority. The authority is to get in there and dig hard on medical conditions. You have to be tenacious. The more you know the residents, the more you'll pick up on something."

As part of their cultural transformation, Veterans Administration nursing homes ask all staff members—nurses, physicians, administrators, secretaries—to help serve food and assist people with eating. "We encourage people to bring their lunches and eat with [residents]," said Christa Hojlo. "The fear is, 'Oh, infection control.' Let's not get hung up—stop looking at the residents as sick hospital patients, but as human beings we're here to serve."

Building Competence

Researcher Barbara Bowers shared with me a cautionary story of a nursing home that prided itself on creating a homey, noninstitutional place to live. A man who lived there became a little confused and was unusually aggressive with other residents. In the old medical model, the first move might be to drug him into submission. Instead, the staff did its best to distract him and to redirect his energy to other activities. But the behavior continued for several weeks. Eventually he collapsed and was admitted to a hospital, where he was diagnosed with bowel cancer. He died soon after. The moral of this true story, said Bowers, is that even as nursing homes strive to transform themselves from hospitals to homes, they still have as a primary responsibility the medical needs of residents.

Steve Shields was reminded of this obligation the year Meadowlark Hills was cited for a number of deficiencies after years with a near-perfect record. One problem the surveyors found was that the staff was growing lax with their hand-washing technique. Reflecting on the survey, Steve said the staff had so embraced the concept of home they had begun to act as you would in your own home. "We had grown too comfortable," he said. "[The surveyors] weren't passing judgment on our model. What they were saying was, 'Yeah, what you're doing is critically important, but you've got to do your fundamental standards of practice. You have to be religious about hand washing.' And they're right."

A series of studies by Better Jobs, Better Care, a $15.5 million, four-year initiative directed by researcher Robyn Stone, found that improving the training and competence of aides is both sorely needed and critical to improving job satisfaction and keeping workers in the field.

But aides are often denied not only the time but also the proper training to make them truly competent. Take the task of helping people eat. Numerous studies have shown a significant number of people in nursing homes— from 35 to 85 percent—are malnourished, making it "one of the largest silent epidemics in this country," according to one study by longtime gerontological nursing researchers.[26] In fact, such experts say, the level of malnutrition and dehydration in some nursing homes is comparable to that found in poverty-stricken developing countries. Improper nutrition is associated with a host of other problems, including increased risk of infections, pressure sores, anemia, low blood pressure, confusion, decreased wound healing, and hip fractures. Not surprisingly, those who lack adequate nutrition are likely to die much sooner than well-nourished nursing home residents.

Helping very old or disabled people to eat is both an art and a skill. Many residents have a condition called dysphagia—difficulty in swallowing—due to a stroke, Alzheimer's disease, or other physical or mental impairment. They are twenty times more likely to develop pneumonia from aspirating food than are people who can eat by themselves.[27] There are ways to help people with dysphagia safely eat. But in many nursing homes, harried, poorly trained aides essentially force-feed residents, shoveling food into their mouths as quickly as possible to get the task done.

Changing the culture of a nursing home is not only about "frills" such as having a cup of Earl Grey tea at sunrise or getting a whirlpool bath rather than a shower. It is also about such basics as getting enough nourishment in a pleasant, dignified manner. Studies show that even such simple things as staff or volunteers greeting residents by name and having normal conversations with them can make a difference in how people eat. In fact, homes that have transformed their culture follow as a matter of course many of the suggestions studies make for improving nutrition. An article in the journal *Contemporary Long Term Care* suggested encouraging weight gain by "creating an environment conducive to eating, including the provision of homelike surroundings at mealtime, smaller social neighborhoods, attractive food, choice in food, attention to ethnically sensitive/appropriate food choices, and making foods available 24 hours a day."[28] The article also suggested cross-training employees throughout the nursing home, including those in administration, to be able to help at mealtime, and recruiting volunteers to socialize.

The workforce crisis in caregiving, along with the culture-change movement, has spawned innovative programs to improve skills and empower aides. The Wellspring model, for example, sends staff teams from different departments and different nursing homes for special training in a given area, such as nutrition or reducing falls. The entire workforce continually hones its skills in a collaborative manner.

"They make sure everyone is on the same page," said Mary Jo Westphal, an aide and care-delivery specialist at a Wisconsin nursing home that used the Wellspring model. "Titles don't matter, to a certain extent. Communication between line staff and dietary and activities, and nurses to CNAs, has completely changed. You never feel belittled when you ask a question. Nurses will ask CNAs questions. We are the eyes for them. We're constantly learning something new. Before, they didn't push education for CNAs or housekeeping. Now the whole line staff learns things at the same time. Everyone has the resident in mind." Even the social barriers were disappearing, she said.

In the past, nurses and aides would not sit at the same table during breaks. But that had changed.[29]

Similarly, LEAP: Learn, Empower, Achieve, Produce, created by the Mather LifeWays Institute on Aging, in Evanston, Illinois, works with aides and nurses to improve skills and raise job satisfaction. Judah Ronch, a psychologist and culture-change expert, was hired in 2005 to improve the quality of nursing homes at Erickson Retirement Communities. Ronch said that after he had introduced LEAP to the staff, "it was very rewarding—not only the change in the way care is provided, but how personally transformative the experience was for them. They changed how they view themselves for the better. People talked about becoming more flexible, more patient, more forgiving, less concerned with routine, and more concerned with quality of life of residents, less centered on their job, and more focused on the experience of the resident. That was one of the great outcomes of the LEAP program."

Enter the Shahbazim

Rena Reid was an eleven-year veteran of nursing homes when I met her in Tupelo, Mississippi. For ten of those years, she worked as a nurse's aide in the traditional nursing home, Cedars, at Traceway, a Methodist continuing-care retirement community. But for the past year, Rena had been one of a select group of aides specially trained to work in the nation's first Green House, a new model of eldercare developed by Bill and Jude Thomas. Four Green Houses had been built on the Traceway campus as a pilot project.

As Bill Thomas writes in *What Are Old People For?*: "The opportunity here is to transform the *dream* of a warm, loving, nurturing sanctuary into a specific *innovation* that can change how we age" (emphasis his).[30] Drawing on models such as monasteries, where unrelated people live together cooperatively, the Green House vision is of an intentional community for people who need supportive services. The Green House is perhaps best known for redesigning the physical layout of a large institution into a cluster of group homes (see the next chapter). But just as important is its reimagining of the role of caregivers. The Green House has upended the management pyramid.

Rena and other aides, now called *shahbazim,* are responsible for running the household on behalf of the elders. A *shahbaz* combines the traditional role of direct caregiver with that of a homemaker and companion to the ten to twelve elders who live in the house. Bill Thomas likes to think of them as "midwives of elderhood" who possess a deep understanding and appreciation of people in the later stage of life.

When I visited the first Green Houses in 2004, the shahbazim had been on the job for a year. Rena's household, like the other Green Houses, was clean, tranquil, and cheerful. Residents spent time in their own private rooms or hung out in common areas, visiting with the staff or singing to themselves.

The serenity was all the more striking after touring Cedars, which was still operating on the campus. The environment there was noisier and tenser. One man draped only in a sheet was being wheeled in a chair to the shower room. He looked frightened. Two aides I interviewed said they were responsible for twenty residents; Rena and another shahbaz care for ten. The aides were in training to be shahbazim, and they were looking forward to more Green Houses opening at Traceway.

Rena said that when she first heard the job title "shahbaz," it seemed strange. According to Bill Thomas, who came up with the term, "shahbaz" means "royal falcon" in Persian. (When I asked if there were no words in the English language to convey what he envisioned, he told me no.) Bill, who is fond of myth and storytelling, invented a legend involving a royal falcon rescuing a wise king who is in trouble. Interestingly, when Traceway advertised for CNAs to come work in an innovative setting, they received only two applications; when they repeated the ad, calling the position a "shahbaz," they received seventy.

Whether or not she feels like a royal falcon, Rena, a soft-spoken woman, seemed to wear the mantle of a shahbaz with pride. As we talked, she puttered around the kitchen with a proprietary air. On the counter were bowls of fruit, chips, a layer cake, and a cookie jar. Part of her training includes cooking; many of the young women grew up on fast food and had few culinary skills before becoming shahbazim. Rena kept a watchful eye on Mrs. Adams, who was finishing her meal at her own slow pace.

To become a shahbaz, Rena explained, "we went through all kinds of training. We learned how to deal with emotional people, how to deal with stress, with someone passing. It's amazing what you can learn." They took courses in cardiopulmonary resuscitation, first aid, and safe lifting techniques, as well as in coping with transition. "We learned how to deal with anger and depression—other people's and our own."

At first, some aides found it difficult to imagine running the household without a nurse there to oversee things. But a team of professionals—nurses, therapists, a physician, a social worker, and a chaplain—is readily available to bring their services to the Green House as needed, rather than having the elders shuttled to them.

Rena and the other shahbazim rotate leadership jobs, such as food coordinator, scheduling coordinator, and housekeeping coordinator. For their extra training and responsibility, shahbazim are paid an additional two dollars an hour, bringing their average hourly wage to ten dollars—not high, but considered a good salary by many in northern Mississippi.

The Green Houses got off to a bumpy start, said Steve McAlilly of Mississippi Methodist Senior Services. "The first weekend we opened, the shahbazim were so focused on cooking, the house could have burned down and they wouldn't have noticed," he joked. "I said, 'Oh, no, what can we use these buildings for?' It's like we were riding a bike without training wheels—you go from wobbly to going with hands in the air and a big smile on your face. I'm not saying it's perfect—it will never be perfect. But challenges a year ago that were mountains are now molehills." Challenges, he said, such as cooking for twelve people three times a day, or "forming teams that truly trust one another."

"Empowerment" is an overworked word, but Rena described what it meant to her: "You don't have nobody pressuring you. Clinical support is not over us. They come in and give meds and see if there's a problem. We do everything except give pills. At Cedars, they told you what you were going to do, and you'd do it or you'd get written up. We have nurses who don't want to come down here [to the Green House] because they can't rule. It feels more like partners now instead of bosses. You've got more time to spend with the elders and with what they need."

As with many aides I interviewed at transformational homes, Rena described her work as "fun." "I like coming to work every day," she said, smiling. "I can be off two days, and the elders will say, 'Where you been?' I'll say, 'I've been off,' and they'll say, 'You've got to quit that.'" She was clearly proud of the affection the residents felt for her. A nurse later told me that on her days off, Rena sometimes visits the sister of a resident who died, "just to be nice."

"One of the things I love is the shahbazim," said Steve McAlilly. "They have become these amazing professional people. I think [before] they were stuck in jobs that were too small for them."[31]

When I visited the Green Houses, I was impressed not only with the shahbazim, but with the nurses and the camaraderie they shared with everyone in the household. They seemed to have time not only to give medications and charting, as all nurses must do, but also to joke around, sing hymns, help unload groceries, assist residents with eating—one was even giving a resident a manicure. The nurses appeared to seamlessly weave their medical duties into the everyday life of the household.

"You really get to be a nurse again instead of running things," said registered nurse Glenda Buchanan, a Green House guide who helps lead the culture-change effort. "It's amazing what the elders teach me—about plants, about life. They miss you when you've been gone. I love it. And it's a joy to watch the shahbazim grow and really take charge."

Shahbazim Code of Ethics

A shahbaz will work with each other as a respectful,
    supportive, flexible team.
A shahbaz will keep their word.
A shahbaz is dependable, honest and trustworthy.
A shahbaz continues to grow, learn and commit to the well-
    being of elders.
A shahbaz includes elders in the decision making as much as
    possible.
A shahbaz never crosses the line between providing care and
    providing clinical treatment.
A shahbaz is patient with elders, each other, and all members
    of the organization and community who come to the
    Green House.
A shahbaz is a good communicator.
A shahbaz shows responsibility to the elders and the other
    members of the team by practicing good work habits
    including:
    Coming in when scheduled and being on time
    Completing their work
    Leaving personal problems at home
    Giving complete reports about the elders
        to the other shahbazim

—Created by the Shahbazim of Tupelo, Mississippi
March 2003

Seeing the Whole Person

Aides, of course, are not just aides. They have full lives outside of work, with families, car problems, bills to pay, churches to attend, and dreams of better things. Recognizing their lives holistically, honoring and encouraging them as people with their own hopes and ambitions and not simply as cogs in the nursing home machine, represents a fundamental piece of a new culture of caring.

At the Mount, employees come from thirty nations. Rather than seeing the cultural and language differences as a problem, staff, managers, family members, and residents told me repeatedly that they enjoyed the diversity. It made life more interesting for all concerned. Steve Ricard, a trim man who was dressed in a bright purple shirt and Mardi Gras beads when I met him—more on Mardi Gras later—described how the Mount was able to keep staff turnover so low. "It's not a glamorous job, so we try to make it a fun work environment," he said.

The Mount goes to great lengths to listen to what the employees want, rather than assuming that management knows best. For example, many employees said they wanted an opportunity to have a home computer, but that they could not afford to buy one. The Mount started a computer loan program, through which it purchases a computer for an employee's home use. The employee has one year to pay for it, at no interest. More than a hundred employees have participated in the program.

Another desire aides around the nation express is a career ladder. Aides at the Mount who want to become nurses can work part-time on the weekends, with some financial assistance, in exchange for a four-year commitment to work there. English-language classes are also available, as is tuition assistance for all kinds of courses. In addition, there is an emergency loan fund for employees who occasionally can't make ends meet, and free gift certificates for food, gas, and bus transportation. As a convenience for employees, on the first Thursday of the month the Mount meal program sells low-cost entrees that feed a family of four. Every other month a local immigrant group—Ethiopian or Filipino, for example—prepares the food. Through its purchase of the prepared meals, the Mount not only gives employees the kind of food they enjoy, but also gives the community a small economic benefit.

For staff and for residents at the Mount, celebrations are big events. There are eight large celebrations a year, such as Mardi Gras; one Christmas the Mount rented a bowling alley for an all-day party and told employees to bring anyone they wanted. Fifteen hundred people came.

Heritage Manor in Lowell also offers a career-development program. Employees have access to tuition reimbursement and grants for getting a high school diploma (GED), English-language classes, nurse training, or other skills at local community college and vocational schools with which Heritage has developed relationships. "We have a career ladder for everybody," said administrator Betty Rozzi. "They help each other through the classes, and their grades are excellent. It's something I like to do—even when they're promoting themselves out of here."

People involved in making nursing homes better places to live and to work describe the process as a journey, never a destination. Using that metaphor, I have observed that the further along the road they are, the more fully empowered the staff—and the better off the residents, whether the measure is quality of health care or the more elusive quality of life. In places I visited, team leaders were chosen not for their efficient bed making, but for their kindness, their creativity, their commitment to treating elders as they would want their own family treated. As the transformation evolves, workers gain the courage to stand up for the residents and for the sacredness of home. In the Green House, for example, the mission of the shahbazim is to "protect, sustain and nurture" the elders in their care. "That gives them the strength to go to the mat when we managers drift back into institutional thinking," said Steve McAlilly.

Rose Marie Fagan, of the Pioneer Network, believes such power sharing is the most important and most difficult change to achieve. At first, she said, managers initiating a change in culture are enthusiastic about trying to honor residents' rights and choices. "When you get to the hard stuff about how power is going to shift, from administrators to people working in the households, that is deep system change," she said. "And it takes skillful leadership and strong and knowledgeable leadership to lead an organization through that process of really transforming an institution into a home."

Chapter 5

"This Is My Home"
Tearing Up the Blueprints

It's hard to speak through and about pain, and it is pain as
well as anxiety, boredom, hope, fatigue, and more that need
to be articulated, concretized, and made into the shape of
a chair, the location of a window, the depth of a sill, the
interior of a toilet stall.
> —Architect Karen Bermann, "Love and Space in the
> Nursing Home"

So much for my family portraits in a room where I can't even
put a thumbtack in the wall.
> —Joyce Horner, *That Time of Year: A Chronicle of Life in
> a Nursing Home*

Before architect David Dillard began redesigning the Village's nursing
home, the staff gave him an assignment. He was to spend twenty-four
hours as a typical resident there. To fully appreciate what people endure, he
was to pretend he had had a stroke, with his right side paralyzed. It was a
challenge for the tall, fit Dillard to keep his right arm and leg limp and immobile, and to ask for help getting in and out of a wheelchair.

"To make matters more interesting, I was supposed to have an eating
condition where everything I ate had to be the consistency of cold cream,"
he said. His colleague, project manager Grant Warner, also took part in the
exercise. He was supposed to have dementia, so he had a "wander guard"
strapped to him that beeped wildly whenever he tried to leave the unit.

The nursing home layout was typical: a wagon wheel, with the nurse's
station at the hub and spokes of long hallways with bedrooms on both sides.
A mix of residents with all sorts of conditions shared the rooms. Dillard's

roommate, "Marlon," had one of the most severe cases of dementia there. "They told me, 'Don't worry, but you may wake up and find him standing over your bed. And he tends to drool.' God bless him, he didn't do it, but the thought of it kept me up until four in the morning," said Dillard. "Plus the sheets were short and I kept feeling the plastic mattress."

His room was also near the nurse's station, a hubbub of activity throughout the night. "It was like being in the first room at the Ramada Inn with the door open all night," he said.

One of many lessons that informed his future design was the simple placement of a light switch. He realized he could not turn his light on and off on his own but had to call for help, making it extremely difficult to read in bed at night.

Bathing was also quite an experience. The bathing room was near the nurse's station, where most residents hung out during the day. Dillard was lifted in a mechanical hoist as the residents and caregivers stared at him. At least, he said, they allowed him to wear bathing trunks.

Navigating a wheelchair one-handed was far more difficult than he had imagined. "At that time, I was a healthy fifty-one-year-old, and I was bumping into people, into doors, into chairs and the furniture. After a few hours, I could see people move away when they saw me coming," he said.

Two images stand out for Dillard. As an afternoon activity, a small band of local musicians performed for residents. Punch and cookies were served. Dillard said he would have enjoyed having cookies, but then he remembered he was not supposed to be able to swallow solid food. More poignant for him, though, was when the musicians invited the residents to join them in playing. Dillard, an accomplished guitar player, very much wanted to participate. He started to volunteer. "But I realized my right arm doesn't work and I couldn't play, as much as I wanted to. The reality of the infirmity set in loud at that moment for me. That stayed with me for a long, long time." He began to more fully appreciate the sense of loss so many nursing home residents feel, not only for their own homes but for much that they love doing.

His most important insight from an architectural standpoint was observing that the residents wanted to be near the staff, no matter how unpleasant the setting. "They had this gigantic nurse's station with broken pink plastic laminate," he said. "There were always eight or twelve residents with their backs to the walls, facing the nurse's station. There were no windows whatsoever, but they parked themselves there. They wanted to physically be close to see their young caretaker friends. I thought there was a major lesson there. What we translated that to is, if the residents are really going to want to be with the caretakers, then let's put the caretakers in wonderful environments, in the corner of a living room, say. Suddenly the whole concept of a nurse's station is blown away."

Dee Dolezal, director of nursing at the Village, recalls the first time she saw the immense nurse's station there. "I was so proud of it," she said. "It was like the *Titanic*."

But after months of rethinking how to make the nursing home like a home, Dee found the nurse's station an embarrassing eyesore. Once the renovation began, she wanted to be the first to raise a sledgehammer.

Smashing the nurse's station is a fitting symbol of the way in which nursing homes transform themselves from a hospital to a home. David Dillard's ordeal as a nursing home resident lasted only a day. Imagine, though, how you would feel living in a hospital-like ward for years on end, confined to half a bedroom, with no privacy; eating every meal off a plastic tray in a cafeteria-like dining hall; negotiating long, slippery hallways; staring at walls that hold nothing of value to you.

Contrast that with Meadowlark Hills or a Green House, places designed like a normal home, with a living room, kitchen, and private spaces to linger.

"We learned early on the household concept was essential," said David Green of Evergreen. "You can't create a home in a bus station. Larger groupings of people do not bring about relationship."

As challenging and expensive as major renovation and construction projects are, the physical transformation of the nursing home is in some ways the simplest change to carry out. Excellent models exist, and the basic building blocks of home are familiar to all of us. Staff members, collaborating with designers, imaginatively deal with what once seemed immutable parts of a nursing home. Large medicine carts, for example, are replaced by small locked medicine cabinets in resident rooms—less efficient for nurses, but far less institutional. Voluminous charts can be electronic, accessible to any computer in the nursing home.

But renovation is also the costliest piece of creating an environment of home. Those who have done it believe the results are well worth the money and effort. Combined with other reforms discussed earlier—resident choice, self-directed staff teams—creating a physical environment of home has a profound effect on residents' well-being.

As have many nursing homes, Fairport Baptist used the opportunity of a needed building renovation to begin the process of culture change. "It is a lot harder without the physical change—it drives the change," said Rev. Garth Brokaw. He described what a difference the first change made: knocking down a large institutional dining room and creating instead three smaller dining areas. "We were trying to feed forty-two dementia folks three times a day at specific times—which doesn't work," he said. "The noise level was incredible, the acting out, the inappropriate behaviors. We were all pulling our hair out trying to figure out how to solve all that and not getting very far."

The smaller dining areas, Garth said, transformed the whole atmosphere for the better. "Overnight, I kid you not, overnight it changed the whole environment on that unit. Just that. The noise level went down." From there, Fairport Baptist created country kitchens, which families and residents use extensively.

As Fairport Baptist discovered, when people see signs of home rather than hospital, the effect can be arresting. Mildred Adams's life was transformed the moment she was wheeled into the nation's first Green House. The transformation was so immediate and seemed so miraculous even Bill Thomas was surprised.

Bill had begun with a simple question. What if, rather than tinker with a hospital design, you created from the ground up a home that would truly meet elders' needs—physically, mentally, emotionally, socially, spiritually?

His answer to that question is the Green House. Green Houses are freestanding homes, not pods or neighborhoods in a large building. They feel like homes and look like homes—albeit homes with ten or so bedrooms. The contrast with Cedars, the traditional large institutional nursing home at Traceway, was sharp. So much so, that Mrs. Adams, who everyone thought was lost in a fog, sat up and took notice.

Mrs. Adams had barely spoken in two years, and her family did not think she recognized them any longer. She had to be spoon-fed pureed food. She was essentially bedridden. In fact, she was not the sort of resident that Traceway wanted to move to the Green House. For the pilot project, they wanted people who were responsive. Mrs. Adams seemed unlikely to survive much longer. But many of the elders at Cedars found change threatening, and they did not want to move. Mrs. Adams's family liked the idea of the Green House and requested that she go there.

"That was a real touching day for us," her daughter-in-law, Becky Adams, said of moving day.

The residents rode over on the Traceway bus. Rena Reid remembers Mrs. Adams's eyes, as soon as she entered the building. She grew more alert, looking around with interest. Rena suggested to the family that they try feeding her at the large dining table with the others.

"My husband was going to feed her," said Becky Adams. "He fed her two bites, and she took the spoon from his hand. She fed herself the rest of the meal. Joni asked her if she wanted a cup of coffee, and she said, 'I believe I will—with a spoon of sugar and a dash of milk.'"

From that first day, Mrs. Adams began singing "Amazing Grace." She soon was back to eating solid food and saying daily blessings. When I met her a year later, she was ninety-four years old and had gained fifteen pounds. "She tells me the food is good," Becky said. "They're not stingy with it! They let them eat at their own pace, and they can eat whenever they want."

Mrs. Adams spoke up. "She's a good cook," she said, nodding toward Rena.

With gentle prompting from Becky, Mrs. Adams agreed to sing some hymns for me. She asked for requests. I said I'd like to hear whatever she was moved to sing. In a sweet, quavery voice she sang "The Old Rugged Cross" and "Amazing Grace."

"I get filled up many a time when I'm singing to myself," she told me.

Asked to what she attributed her mother-in-law's reawakening, Becky said, "It's not a hospital-like facility. I have wondered if she had gotten into a depressed state. Now she's out there where everything is going on. She always liked people and was a leader, and active in her church. At Cedars, she was in a dark drab room or out in the hall. Here, it's more like coming to her home. It's such a contrast. It's giving people a more secure feeling, like they're in a home. We're just so overcome with the place. It makes you not dread full-time care."

Other family members and residents of the Green Houses repeatedly echoed these sentiments. "This is so much better," said Clyde Biddle, whose wife, Sara, in her fifties, was the youngest resident there. "It really is so much more like a home. In Cedars we ate all our meals in the room—we had no interaction with other residents. This is cheaper than a private room at a nursing home. When I walk in, they're cooking and it smells like home. It's so simple a concept, you'd think someone would have thought of it before."

Clyde came daily to eat with the household around the dining table, family style. Having a big dining room table was a fundamental part of the Green House concept—"the one place where the most people sit around and laugh and tell stories and have hard discussions and cry," as Steve McAlilly put it.

Another important feature of the Green Houses—and a rarity in places that depend primarily on Medicaid reimbursement, as Traceway does—is that each resident has a private bedroom and bath. To the Biddles, this privacy gave Sara far more dignity. They could also decorate the room as they wished. She slept in a favorite antique painted-iron bed.

Each bedroom opens onto the common area, called the hearth, to encourage residents to socialize with others in the household. The walls around the hearth of the Franks household (each household was named for the eldest person to first live there) were a deep slate blue, and the comfortable chairs are upholstered in burgundy and blue. A gold-framed mirror hung over the fireplace, and on the mantle were dolls, vases of both real and artificial flowers, a big blue plastic piggy bank, a china vase that said "Washington, D.C.," and philodendrons—a motley assortment, chosen not by a decorator but by those who work and live in the Green House.

During my visit, I saw people enjoying the full space of the Green Houses, inside and out. One woman, who walked through her house in a dreamy state, was always poking her head outside. She twirled an umbrella made of a fabric printed with cats and dogs. "I don't think it's rained since I bought it," she told me. She and others frequently went outdoors to the secure patio, some to smoke cigarettes. Outdoors, each Green House has a small yard with birdfeeders, windchimes, a barbecue grill, and benches. Sara Biddle said she enjoyed being able to sit outside after supper with her husband.

Residents, family members, and staff shared small miracles with me throughout my stay at Traceway. Some residents who had been confined to wheelchairs because they could not manage the long hallways of Cedars were able to walk from their rooms around the entire house.

"The environment creates opportunities and space for life, for living," said Steve McAlilly. "What is it like to struggle across a room rather than be popped in a wheelchair? Struggle is important for life."

Many residents seemed to feel the Green House was a much nicer place than they had ever lived in before. Mrs. Cynthia Dunn spoke with great pride of being there. "This is my home," she said grandly. She and her friend Mrs. Franks enjoyed helping with laundry. "But I don't do ironing," she said, laughing.

Normalcy reigned. I overheard one shahbaz calling another household, asking to borrow ice cream. Another called to ask for an iron, to press a dress for an elder who was going to a funeral. It all seemed so natural, like any close-knit community where a neighbor would borrow a cup of sugar.

Steve McAlilly said he often wondered why it seemed so much easier to provide a high quality of life to people in the Green Houses compared to a traditional nursing home. "I keep coming back to the physical structure," he said. "The environment sets the tone for the culture. This is culture replacement. Culture change is taking an existing structure and trying to change what's going on. Culture replacement is smashing what's there and replacing it." By building from the ground up, Steve believes, you are far less likely to slip back into the old institutional mindset and practices.

The Eden Alternative

In the early 1990s, Bill Thomas was working as a physician in a traditional nursing home in upstate New York when he had a revelation about how life could be made better for people who lived and worked there. "In terms of what we do in long-term care, it's about the most biophobic environment you can imagine," he told me. "Anyone who has spent any time in a nursing home has a sense of destitution in the way the environment is stripped bare of any semblance of the living world. . . . We've taken the metaphor of the operating room with its sterility and gleaming tile and walls and extended it to places it does not belong."

He and his wife, Jude, developed a model based instead on a "human habitat." Called the Eden Alternative, this new approach involves a comprehensive ten-stage process of change (see Appendix C). It is best known for creating an enriched, living environment of plants, pets, and children.

Chase Memorial, the first Eden Alternative nursing home, at one point had eighty parakeets, ten finches, two lovebirds, half-a-dozen cockatiels, two canaries, two dogs, four cats, and an assortment of rabbits and chickens. In place of a lawn was a garden of peas, beans, squash, melons, spinach, corn and other vegetables for the residents to enjoy.

A growing body of research shows the salubrious effects of being around animals, houseplants, and nature. Roger Ulrich of Texas A&M University has designed experiments that demonstrate how views of nature affect hospital patients, prisoners, and office employees. In study after study, he and others have shown that even a picture of trees or water can help lower blood pressure and decrease muscle tension. Patients who view nature reportedly have less pain and shorter hospital stays than their counterparts without such a view.[1]

Planetree, in its patient-centered approach, works with architects to soften and enrich hospitals with "healing gardens," fountains, and paintings of nature. In the same way, nursing homes install aquariums and aviaries to soothe patients who have dementia. Even before Bill Thomas's Eden Alternative, nursing homes such as Teresian House in Albany, New York, encouraged staff to regularly bring pets to work.

Over time, some three hundred nursing homes in the United States and two hundred more around the world have become Eden-certified, sending key staff members for training and committing to the Eden goals. Nevertheless, the institutional feel still dominates at many of these homes. In the worst cases, some nursing homes appeared to do little more than buy a few parakeets or philodendrons and declare themselves Edenized, rather than doing the hard work of building community. After ten years of working to recreate nursing homes through the Eden Alternative, Bill Thomas became convinced that change wasn't happening as quickly or as deeply as he had imagined.

He decided the best way to uproot the institutional nature of nursing homes was to begin from the bottom up. The Green House would be the Eden Alternative made real. He began to call himself an abolitionist. "One down, seventeen thousand to go," he cheerfully told me when Traceway decided to do away entirely with its traditional nursing home and create a street of Green Houses instead.

Other nursing homes have created imaginative ways to make not just a household environment but an entire neighborhood. The Mount in Seattle has a lively street scene on the inside walls of its aging building. Saddled with what in-house architect Dyke Turner described as a "horrible infrastructure" of columns and long narrow halls, the Mount came up with a way to build appealing common spaces along a faux Main Street off the lobby.

In keeping with java-loving Seattle, residents, staff, volunteers, and families mingle at the Mount's espresso bar. Robbie, the barista, who looked like a middle-aged rock star, with tight jeans, boots, and a bleached mullet, served up a steady stream of lattes and hot chocolate. The café also has a gift shop with greeting cards, candy, dolls, and fancy soap. Across the "street" are a thrift shop, pharmacy, beauty parlor, and one of the Mount's four day-care centers for children of staff and the larger community. A window cut into the wall of the day-care center allows passersby to watch the children playing. Down the hall is a wellness clinic with massage, acupuncture, chiropractor, podiatrist, and a sewing shop, where volunteers do mending for residents and staff, as well as make clothing to raise money for the Mount's charitable foundation. Residents' and children's art lines the halls. Contributing to the sense of a street scene is a real park bench and street lamp with vines and birds painted on the wall behind.

"The biggest impact we had was providing more common space," said Dyke. "Prior to this, the dining room was the only public space, and the halls and a little bit of activity space. You need common space for people to interact. If you don't, then you don't really have private space either—you have places of isolation instead."

The Nursing Home as a Sensual Experience

The hospital model is a flawed concept not only for nursing homes, but also, as Planetree argues, for acute-care hospital patients. As Ulrich and other researchers have demonstrated, the unpleasant hospital environment has been linked to elevated blood pressure, anxiety, delirium, nausea, increased need for medication, and longer postoperative stays for patients. Planetree advocates engaging the senses of hospital patients in pleasing ways, by reducing such elements as unpleasant noise and introducing features such as music or natural light.

Similarly, architect Ruven Liebhaber of Lexington, Massachusetts, uses a "sensory approach" to design hospice cottages. Traditionally, architects design institutions in a more technical way, he explained—how many air exchanges per hour in the room, for example. He asks different questions: "How am I affected in terms of movement of air across my skin or concentration of smells? What will stimulate my vision? What will feel nice to touch, in terms of where I'm sitting and what the walls are, and how I'm gripping my handrail? It means really examining our five senses as you design the environment."

What could these design ideas mean in the context of a nursing home? Replacing the noise of buzzers and loudspeakers with normal human conversation or music (although people's taste in music, I have observed, is so individual that it is hard to please any group). Replacing the repugnant smells of the worst nursing homes—disinfectant and human waste—with the aroma of baking bread, frying bacon, or flowering plants.

Human touch can be a rare delight for older people, especially those who have no family members nearby. Simply sitting and holding hands with a caregiver or volunteer, or giving and receiving a hug, is deeply comforting. So is stroking a favorite quilt or petting a cat or dog. In his book, former nursing home aide Tom Gass recalled a resident with dementia who was often very anxious. "Somebody came in and set a puppy in her lap," he wrote. "For over an hour, she was totally happy to have this contact, this physical touch. People need that."

In an environment designed to appeal to the senses, meals would be prepared or served in the resident's household rather than in a large commercial kitchen, so that aromas can pique the tastebuds and the food tastes better and fresher. An article in the *Journal of Gerontological Nursing* recommended such simple practices as providing tablecloths and placemats, eliminating serving trays, and seating people at tables of six or eight as ways to make eating more enjoyable.[2]

Visually, a genuine home is a feast for the eyes, compared to a sterile institution. In a resident's room, cherished belongings, family photos, and furniture bring comfort and familiarity. Far too many traditional nursing homes lack even simple amenities such as a shelf in a resident's bedroom. In one nursing home, architect Karen Bermann writes, enterprising staff hung a hammock from the ceiling to hold a resident's large collection of stuffed animals. On the walls throughout a transformed nursing home are pictures of nature, children's drawings, warm colors, all kinds of homey touches that hold meaning for those who live and work there.

The residents' environment extends beyond the walls of the nursing home. People need access to the outside world, whether it's through informal gardens, courtyards, a room with a view of a tree, or fishing ponds. Bigfork Valley Communities has a wheelchair-accessible dock where residents can fish in the Bigfork River. It's a lovely spot, with wild rice growing on the banks and ducks coming in for a landing. The Mount is fortunate to be situated on a hill in West Seattle, overlooking at night the stunning lights of the city skyline and Space Needle. Windows frame views of Mount Rainier or pink-blossomed cherry trees. "The beautiful view is really important to [residents]," said Hipp Tiniacos, an aide at the Mount. "They are afraid of the darkness and seeing nothing in front of them. They want nothing ugly or just walls. They need to see light and to see beautiful things." When residents are troubled or agitated, he sometimes brings them to a window just to gaze out at the mountains.

Bigfork is about as out of the way as you can find in the continental United States. (For some reason, many of the most cutting-edge, innovative nursing homes are off the beaten path.) To get to Bigfork, my husband and I drove through gently rolling hills, passing an occasional bison farm, before we entered the North Woods. At evening, a hazy golden light haloed the tops of the birch trees. It is a quiet world of hunters and fisherfolk, hardy souls who love the crunch of snow, the cry of loons, the soaring bald eagles.

The federal government designated the Bigfork area "medically under-served," meaning it had a shortage of health professionals. Despite being in a poor, rural area with a dearth of workers and funding, the leaders of Bigfork Valley Communities (formerly called Northern Pines) decided in 1997 to take what they described as an "incredible journey" to create "a whole new world for our elders, their families, our staff who care for our elders, and the communities we serve."[3] It was here that Steve Shields had his epiphany of "home."

Just as Meadowlark Hills drew on Bigfork, Bigfork drew on other exemplary homes, such as Evergreen in Oshkosh and the Swedish Service House in St. Paul, to come up with its model. Spruce Lodge, the first transformed household at Bigfork, reflected the local culture and surroundings in its decor. Snowshoes and quilts hung on the walls. In the hall was a comfortable loveseat with a tree-branch motif. Images of pine trees and mallard ducks patterned fabrics of forest green.

In the living room, I visited with a group of residents who had gathered around a warm fire after breakfast. It was a cozy scene. Pale sunlight came through a bay window. A golden retriever, Goldie, with a yellow bow tucked behind her ear, lay with her head on her paws. Wilfred, a white cat, walked by.

"Goldie is my sweetheart," said one woman. "I've had her for many years."

Another woman commented on how well the staff took care of the animals. "How do you have time?" she asked no one in particular.

"They do a lot for us—and for the animals," offered another.

A voice of pessimism—or perhaps pragmatism—chimed in. "You'd be crazy to say you love it here," she said. "I loved taking care of myself. But you have to accept it."

I grew accustomed to these voices, the mix of cheerfulness and stoicism, light and dark, determination and resignation. Transformation is not a magic elixir. Residents will always face trials and losses. But every place I visited held stories of hope.

The Spruce Lodge staff credited Wilfred, the cat, with saving the life of a determinedly solitary resident. In the traditional nursing home, the woman believed everyone was poisoning her. She refused to eat and so was tube fed. After moving to Spruce Lodge, she gradually emerged from her paranoia. She became attached to Wilfred. She began eating and showing up for social events. "It's home, community, and relationships" that made the difference, said Carla, the community coordinator for Spruce Lodge.

Another resident, "Mr. Williams," had been one of the most ornery residents of the nursing home. Suffering from serious vascular disease, he had arrived in a wheelchair, determined to prove that he would be ill-treated. He lined up three urinals and focused every day on getting staff to empty them as frequently and promptly as possible. His favorite pastime was pushing his call light and carefully timing the response. If the time exceeded what he felt was reasonable—say, five minutes—he called the state long-term care ombudsman and filed a complaint.

Carla recalled what happened when they told Mr. Williams he had been chosen to move into the remodeled household from the old nursing home wing. "We were just beginning to get a sense of the new construction. We brought him in and told him he could pick his room. He burst into tears. He said, 'This is a nursing home? I get to live here? I get to pick my room?' He started talking about where he would put his things."

After the move, said Carla, "he began to play music again, he had a harmonica. He came back to life. He started leading Bible study. We moved in in October. On New Year's Eve, he joined the community band. He thrived. He liked jalapeno peppers on everything!"

Mr. Williams had died six months before my arrival, so I couldn't hear the story from him. But Carla attributed his rejuvenation in part to the control and privacy he regained through having his own room. "He got to continue life in a positive way," she said, "instead of focusing on the call light and the urinals and the clock."

The staff shared many stories that demonstrated the power of home. One resident had been a cook in a logging camp. After Bigfork built a family-style kitchen, she sometimes would arise at two o'clock AM to make caramel rolls, with the help of an aide. Everyone would be invited to the household later in the morning for coffee and fresh-baked rolls.

Owning the Design

No matter how lovely the furnishings or how well conceived the architectural drawings, a nursing home will not feel comfortable unless those who live and work there have a sense of ownership. "There are ones where the director of nursing decorated, and it's lovely, but nobody who uses it feels any different about the environment," said Pam Elrod of Genesis. "But the administration is very proud to show you—'Look at our beautiful bathing environment, now my residents have a better place to bathe.' But the residents and staff don't take pride in keeping it up. It's not theirs. They don't own it. I'm not sure any feel any more pleasure being hoisted into the tub than they would have. That's not really culture change—it's a prehistoric, primal version compared to a very sophisticated, visceral success."

At Meadowlark Hills, the dietary staff helped design the kitchens in the households, and the aides designed the bathrooms.

At Fairport Baptist, a lovely modern stained-glass window designed by residents and staff graces the chapel. "The residents didn't want an old-style stained-glass or an abstract design," said Rev. Garth Brokaw. "They wanted a window that said who we are as a Baptist home." The window includes images of a wheelchair, a walker, and pets among scenes that represent the home's religious heritage. A banner in the chapel reads: "Serving the aging who shaped our heritage."

Architect Martin Siefering of Perkins Eastman in Pittsburgh explains how including aides in culture change has an impact on the design process. "A lot of the best knowledge lies with the front-line staff," he said. "Bathing a resident is a pretty intimate thing. When you talk to a CNA about how they get a resident who has some mobility issues up and out of bed to a shower chair, how to deal with incontinence in the bathroom, you can make the design of the bathroom better—making sure there are plenty of towels in reach, if they need to keep someone warm. It's those intimate details that make a better experience."

One challenge is that most nursing home employees have never before read architectural drawings. Siefering and his colleagues use cardboard boxes to build a full-size mockup of a bathroom. The aides can get a better sense of the plans and make sure there is space to move a wheelchair, for example. One of the frustrations of many older nursing homes is that they were built in a time when few residents used wheelchairs, unlike today when most residents do.

Ruven Liebhaber suggests nursing homes could be designed in the same way as hospice cottages. In his designs, Liebhaber involves as many people as possible, including family members, volunteers, and staff. Together, they suggest features that will make family and friends feel comfortable and at home. "Having all of those people involved in the project and feel they've had a meaningful part in it helps in a multitude of ways," he said. "So the same thing can be for nursing homes, if the planning is more community based, rather than just imposed. That would make a very big difference."

When a House Is Not a Home

A nursing home environment that looks like home is tremendously powerful. But it is not powerful enough on its own to provide nursing home residents a high quality of life. Even the most homey-looking place can be deceiving. While in Kansas, I heard of a place described by its owner as a Green House. At that time, the only Green Houses were in Tupelo, so I was curious. I called to arrange for a visit.

Located in a residential neighborhood in a small town, the house was a modest rambler that served as a group home for three women who qualified for skilled nursing care. A young aide in a smock and slacks greeted me at the front door. She asked me to sit in the silent living room. The sound of a television carried from a back room.

Eventually I was escorted back to see "Mrs. Anderson," a registered nurse who owned the operation. Her three charges were finishing up supper. They sat around the small dining table and ate in silence, then wheeled themselves into their bedrooms for the night. It was only about six o'clock on a beautiful end-of-summer day. But it seemed it was their bedtime. Mrs. Anderson ran a tight ship.

She had gotten wind of the Green House concept, but the only thing that registered in her mind was that it was a small-scale group home, which she felt she offered. To me the home seemed contaminated by the mindset of a large institution.

I asked Mrs. Anderson what she thought of the idea of nursing home residents setting their own schedules. "Oh, no, I wouldn't agree with that at all," she said, shaking her head firmly. "That might be all right for assisted living, but not for skilled nursing care."

I pressed her on it. To her, honoring residents' preferences amounted to "spoiling" them. The important thing was that she and her assistant be able to run their little operation smoothly—what was convenient for them easily trumped the residents' desires (even though the residents were paying a princely sum for their long-term care).

I asked whether the women could choose what they wanted to eat, or if they might help in the kitchen to the best of their abilities. I had noticed a gate barred the way to the kitchen. Again, the firm shake of the head. "I don't want them messing around my kitchen. They might get hurt. They might spill something, or get burned on the stove, or break a glass," Mrs. Anderson said.

I thought of Ida at Meadowlark, who wanted a cup of Earl Grey at sunrise in a Staffordshire china cup. She would surely be out of luck here.

Homemaking on a Budget

Most nursing homes are likely to say they cannot afford the multimillion-dollar construction projects described here. The for-profit nursing homes that make up the vast majority are especially at a disadvantage in raising money for improvements; nonprofit homes can solicit tax-free donations for capital campaigns. A nonprofit's board of directors may also be more supportive than faceless shareholders might be. At Meadowlark Hills, for example, Steve Shields has a board of directors who live in the community and take pride that their nursing home is exemplary. Nursing homes owned by large for-profit corporations may have a tough time convincing shareholders who live thousands of miles away that investing in renovations at a particular nursing home is worthwhile. Small privately owned homes may simply not have the funds.

But even facilities unable to undertake substantial renovation can create a more inviting environment. Those with enthusiastic and committed staff are taking steps to approximate home as best they can.

Heritage Manor in Lowell, Massachusetts, is a modest structure. Many of the residents come from poor backgrounds, including a few who lived on the streets of the old mill town before ending up in the nursing home.

But under the leadership of administrator Betty Rozzi, Heritage Manor strives to make meaningful change, even in the design of the home. When Heritage first began its culture-change journey, the staff watched a Pioneer Network video of Steve Shields and life at Meadowlark Hills. The staff was both excited and skeptical that Heritage Manor could ever be like that. "Seeing that video, my first impression was, look at that building. No way it will happen here. It was a great idea, but—never happen. Then we challenged ourselves to not worry about aesthetics and do what we could to give residents more choices," said Andy Andreopoulos, the director of nursing at that time.

"To be perfectly honest, three years ago, I thought there's no way it could happen in an old building," agreed Tracy, the youthful dietary director, who gave me a tour. "I put all the negatives out there."

When I visited, they had made progress. With some extra money in the budget, the staff transformed a room into a bright country kitchen that can accommodate eighteen residents at a time. In the mornings, the staff serves up bacon, eggs, pancakes, and English muffins. "Steps, little steps, that's what we take to make culture change," was Tracy's mantra.

Families had seldom used another large room, designated the family room, preferring the sunnier lobby instead. The staff thought the space might be put to better use as a game room, with a pool table, Tracy explained, and "we asked the residents what they would prefer." When the idea was presented to residents at their monthly council meeting, they liked the idea. A pool table donated by a staff member was now in the room. On the walls hung sports memorabilia and baseball caps, also donated by staff. Puzzles and games were stacked on shelves. When a major sports event is aired, residents and staff drag in chairs, and everyone gathers to eat popcorn and enjoy it together.

The staff was planning to knock down the nurse's station in the Alzheimer's wing next. Unlike some newer places that have wandering paths for those with dementia, at Heritage, residents trudged back and forth in the halls, squeezing past carts. The hope was to open up the nurse's station, making it a common area for staff and residents, with no boundary between them. I asked a nurse what she thought of the idea. She said she liked it in theory, to make the wing feel homier, but she was worried how it would affect her work. How would she be able to complete the painstaking work of filling out government-required assessment forms if people with dementia were constantly interrupting? she wondered. But she was willing to give it a try.

Heritage had added other small touches. Local school children had painted a bright nature scene on the walls, and staff had done their best to transform a basement lounge into a tropical paradise, with a life-size photomural of the ocean and palm trees covering one wall, and another wall painted with tropical fish. "Steps, little steps," Tracy repeated.

When I asked Betty Rozzi what Heritage Manor will look like in twenty years, she said she hoped they will have a new building, one that better reflects their resident-centered mission.

The first thing I saw when I pulled up to another Genesis-owned home, Ridgewood in Bedford, New Hampshire, was a pine grove, with picnic tables scattered under the trees. The day was windy and cold, with icy puddles. But I could easily imagine how pleasant it would be in warm weather to sit in the grove and enjoy a picnic.

Off the main lobby was a large, comfortable parlor with an organ, book-shelves, and a fireplace, with the dining room beyond.

"We're planning to open the dining room from eleven o'clock to eight and offer room service, like a restaurant," said culture-change leader and aide Theresa Smith. "It's still not home, but it would be less institutional and more like a nice hotel."

Ridgewood had institutional hallways and small shared bedrooms. But for one floor, "Corporate" had allocated funds to build a new bathing suite. Residents would not have to travel down such a long hallway from their rooms to be bathed, giving them more privacy and dignity. A bedroom was being "decommissioned" to accommodate the new suite, and the subsequent loss of income, said Theresa, was most unusual and represented to her Genesis's commitment to their efforts.

Regulators Run Amok

Cost is the biggest barrier to redesigning nursing homes, but regulators also can burden the process toward change. Architect David Hoglund of Perkins Eastman explains that most states' Medicaid programs will reimburse nursing homes for construction costs, but only up to a point. Reimbursements for capital improvements can be so low that they compel nursing homes to limit the amount of space devoted to residents. "In some states this actually translates to a maximum square footage per bed," says Hoglund. "This maximum is for the total facility, meaning bedroom, corridor, dining, offices, activity rooms and so on. These limits are typically in a low range that would make it virtually impossible to do all or nearly all private rooms."

As architect Benyamin Schwarz explains in *Nursing Home Design: Consequences of Employing the Medical Model*, well-intentioned architects are sometimes stymied in their efforts at creative home design. Schwarz interviewed state regulators, architects, and nursing home owners about the plan-approval process. He demonstrated how regulatory agencies pushed nursing home operators away from innovation. Some state codes restricted a room size to a degree that hampered residents' autonomy and independence, especially that of people in wheelchairs. In one remarkable interview Schwarz conducted, a state regulator said of resident bedrooms:

Several years ago, we began to receive some applications from people who wanted to build 300–400 sq. ft. for a room. Their idea was for a nursing home patient to be able to bring furniture in and make that room a *home* [emphasis his] rather than just make a patient room. We said well, if a patient in a nursing home is that sick the patient probably doesn't need any furniture, doesn't want that furniture. And besides we don't want that person to become isolated in their room. We like to see that person get out of the room and into an activity room where that person can socialize.[4]

Because of such thinking, residents are still stuck in unlivable places. Reform leader Carter Williams described a woman who lived in a constant state of frustration due to two small features of her environment. The woman, who had emphysema, got around in a wheelchair. She had always been a clotheshorse and had in her bedroom in the nursing home a closetful of custom-made fashions that she dearly loved. But her room was so small that she could not maneuver her wheelchair around to have access to her clothes. In addition, she was unable to reach her toiletries: Aides trying to tidy the bathroom kept moving them out of reach. On constant rotation, the aides could not possibly remember and honor her wishes.[5]

Christa Hojlo of the VA nursing homes said strict fire regulations also get in the way of making places feel more like home. "I've had facilities where residents helped fix up the hallways, just to have facilities management take it all down," she said. "A fire chief said to me, 'There's nothing worse than dying in a fire.' I said, 'Yes, there is—dying in a nursing home, in restraints, in an environment where my humanity is totally undressed.' I'd rather die fast in a fire than be waiting to die in an environment that is horrific." (She added that VA nursing homes have sprinklers, evacuation plans, and highly skilled emergency personnel to deal with fires.)

Nursing home leaders willing to be proactive on behalf of elders involve regulatory and safety staff early in the renovation or construction process, explaining their goals and how their design will achieve them.

In the future, new technology developed for people with disabilities will open up all sorts of possibilities for nursing homes. Already, at many homes, staff use beepers and cell phones and are no longer tethered to a central nurse's station, hardwired to the call lights over residents' rooms.

Oatfield Estates, an innovative assisted-living community outside Portland, Oregon, combines handsome residential homes, organic gardens, and spectacular mountain views with the latest technology to keep residents safe. The community is made up of large two-story houses, each with ten private bedrooms and baths, plenty of windows, and open common areas for dining, watching television, cooking, and socializing. Young culinary school graduates act as personal chefs for each household, and a few employees even live there. Residents are free to help themselves in the kitchen.

Oatfield uses a sophisticated computer monitoring system that may be the wave of the near future. Through electronic sensors, the staff can tell when a person at risk of falling gets out of bed. The system can be programmed to automatically turn on low lights at night to show the way to the bathroom, or to automatically turn off a stove if a person with memory loss comes near it. Residents have complete freedom to go outdoors and walk around the lovely grounds; there are no locks or fences. Those with dementia wear a badge that discreetly signals the staff if they start to leave the property. New technology such as this opens up wonderful possibilities for people to be independent and safe, whether they remain in their own homes or move to a group setting.

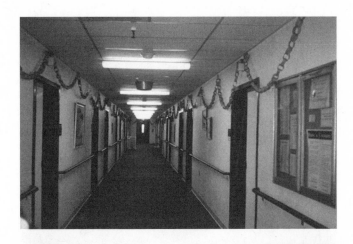

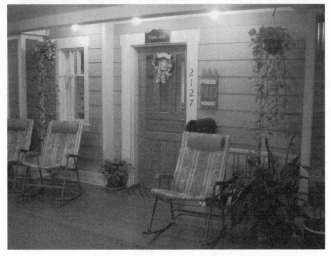

Before its transformation, Meadowlark Hills in Manhattan, Kansas, had a typical nursing home with long hospital corridors. (Courtesy of Meadowlark Hills.) Today, this is the scene that greets you as you enter Ptacek House, a resident household. (Photo by Jeff Chapman.)

Helen Wendling and Maxine "Micky" Worster help cook a meal in the Lyle household at Meadowlark Hills. (Photo by Jeff Chapman.)

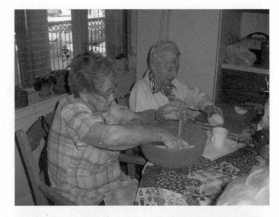

Ruth Reid brought her sewing machine when she moved to Meadowlark Hills, and she continues to enjoy making quilts. (Photo by Jeff Chapman.)

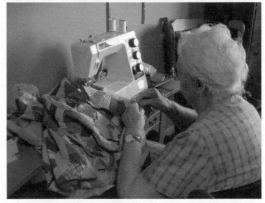

In transformative homes, residents are encouraged to help with everyday chores if they wish, such as selecting menus and preparing food, doing personal laundry, or taking care of pets and plants. Making a contribution is one way to counter what Dr. Bill Thomas calls the three plagues of nursing home life: loneliness, helplessness, and boredom.

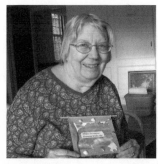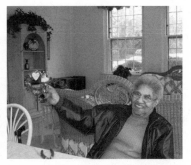

Jacki Kelly and Jean Pierce show artwork they created while
making the transition to assisted living at the Lisner-Louise-
Dickson-Hurt Home in Washington, D.C. (Photos by Karen
Gallant.)

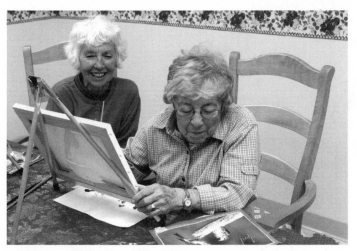

At Wesley Village in Shelton, Connecticut, residents have
many opportunities for creativity and self-expression. Jackie
McDougall, *left*, watches as Margaret Jacaruso works on a
painting. (Photo by Skip Hine.)

New research shows that old age can be a fertile time for
creativity, even for those who have never pursued artistic work
before or who have dementia.

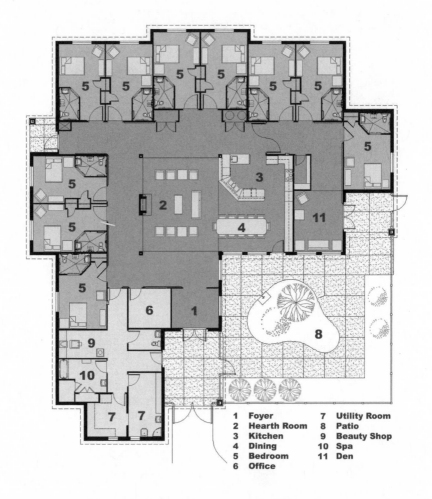

1	Foyer	7	Utility Room
2	Hearth Room	8	Patio
3	Kitchen	9	Beauty Shop
4	Dining	10	Spa
5	Bedroom	11	Den
6	Office		

The floor plan of a Green House: Every resident has a private bedroom and bath, and all rooms open to the common area to encourage camaraderie. (Copyright 2003 The McCarty Company.)

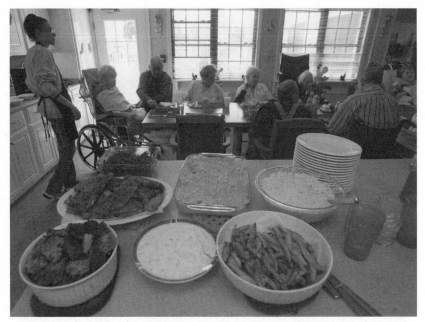

At Green Houses, residents eat family style. Fresh home-cooked food is always available, and elders eat at their own pace. *Below:* Dale Letson, a Green House shahbaz in Tupelo, Mississippi, says cooking is one of the things she enjoys most about her job. Shahbazim combine the roles of homemaker, caregiver, and friend to residents. (Courtesy of Mississippi Methodist Senior Services.)

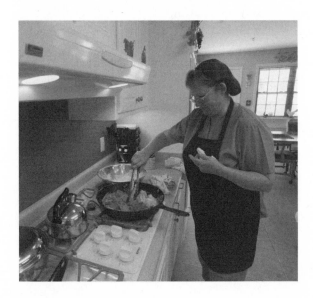

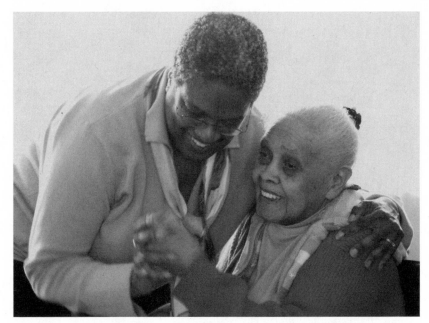

Transformative homes are welcoming to families. Frances Biner and her daughter cut a rug at Buchanan Place in Seattle, as part of "Unleashed Memory," a cross-generational project of the Next Stage Dance Theatre. The project demonstrates how people with memory loss can benefit from dance and music. (Photo by Robert E. Kittilson.)

Chapter 6

"You Can Dance Alone or We'll Dance with You"

Creating Community

We're so schedule driven now. We can't have a relationship
with the residents—to get forty-four people up, dressed, to
breakfast, to the bathroom—there's no time.
> —Dee Dolezal, director of nursing, the Village,
> before culture change

What touches my heart is to know the elders in their winter
years will actually have a home. Some of these people, we're
the only family they have. It is exciting to wake up and come
to work every day. What more could you want? I'm ready to
step out in faith.
> —Glenda Buchanan, registered nurse
> and Green House guide

These are the happiest years of our lives.
> —Phillip Bellefeuille, ninety-five,
> on living with his wife, Alean, at the Mount

When I first entered Providence Mount Saint Vincent in Seattle, Mardi
Gras was in full swing. A Dixieland band was swaying in the lobby, and
plenty of folks, young and old, were gathered around, some in wheelchairs,
all tapping to the beat.

From the outside, the Mount looks rather imposing. A 300,000-square-
foot brick edifice, constructed in 1924 for the Sisters of Providence (who now
live in an adjacent building), the Mount offers assisted living and a nursing
home for people of all faiths. It may not be the most modern, elegant, or
homelike in its bricks and mortar, but in fifteen years of "resident-directed"
culture, the Mount has forged a deep sense of community.

On a tour, I glimpsed images of real life. Coming down the hall was a young woman, dressed in t-shirt and jeans, pulling a large plastic wagon that carried three round-cheeked babies solemnly watching the world go by. The Mount has four onsite day-care centers, and children are a regular feature of daily life. A group of older men strolled through the halls crooning "Cajun Love Song," while a woman walking with them rolled her eyes and indicated with a twirl of her finger that they were crazy. Family members, volunteers, and residents shopped for treasures in the thrift shop or sat in the espresso bar having coffee. I heard laughter and conversation. No one wore uniforms (the result of a request by residents). The Mount seemed to be achieving its goal of "normalcy" for people who live there.

The highlight of Mardi Gras week was a parade of staff, family members, and residents, each with a dog in costume: a shih tzu dressed as a nun, a Yorkshire terrier in red plaid, a miniature dachshund with a red feathered mask, a homely old mutt with a big underbite and a baseball cap, another dachshund in a baby bonnet, cocooned in a quilt. I followed the parade as it snaked its way through the building. Most of the residents seemed delighted, although a few looked confused. The hilarity was contagious, though. Celebrations such as this are frequent, I was told. Any occasion will do, even Oprah's birthday. Cathy Butler, sixty-one, a younger resident with lifelong disabilities, would later tell me, "And parties! Do we know how to party! We'll open a bottle of champagne at the drop of a hat." She filled me in on the latest cocktail, a poinsettia, made with champagne and cranberry juice. "That's what we drank on Super Bowl Sunday," she said. Cathy said her life was fuller since she'd moved to the Mount, and she had a wide circle of friends.

Kathryn Anderson taught nursing students for twenty years before she became director of nursing at the Mount in 2005. She said she realized in those two decades the only mornings that she woke up eager to come to work were the days when she was bringing students to the Mount for a geriatric rotation. "I felt happy just coming through the doors," she said.

Happiness and fun—in such short supply in so many nursing homes—seemed abundant here. I spoke with Penny Garrett, an aide who had worked on and off at the Mount since 1986. She, like many of her coworkers, was from the Philippines. She had worked at other nursing homes in Seattle and in Georgia, and she believed the community at the Mount was special. "Some other places, people don't talk and laugh, and the residents worry. It's depressing. You got more load, not enough help, and the staff become frustrated. Here, what I see, you know everybody. Even if you wake up on the wrong side of the bed—here we're cracking up for nothing. Just to say good morning is fun. Here you can talk among each other. If I have a harder group [of residents], with someone sick, the others will help me."

I visited Penny on the third-floor "neighborhood" where she worked.

Residents, arriving at their own pace for breakfast, sat at small dining tables. Country music was on the radio. Penny said they stopped having television on because many people became so mesmerized with the screen they forgot to eat. The room is long and narrow. At one end was a desk and computer where the nurses do their charting. In the middle was the dining area, and at the other end a home-sized kitchen. Most people sat quietly, although one woman repeated in a low voice what sounded like, "Please tell me, please tell me."

As part of its shift to resident-directed care and normalcy, the Mount went from seventeen special diets to four. On the tables are salt and pepper shakers, sugar bowls, and bottles of hot sauce. A nurse said she was surprised when visitors touring from another nursing home were as impressed by these condiments as by anything else; in their facility such seasonings were strictly controlled.

Penny served a table of four men, whom she obviously knew well. To one she said, "I put a lot of brown sugar in your oatmeal, so taste it before you add more sugar." He picked up his spoon and smiled kindly at Penny. "You're a good girl," he told her.

I asked Penny if she ever cooked Filipino food for residents. Yes, she said, chicken and rice, eggrolls, and *pancit*, a noodle dish. "Some don't care for it, but the majority like it," she said.

Once the residents were settled into breakfast, Penny and I walked down the hall for a chat. She said she was having a difficult week and felt "double sad." Two people had died—Bob, a longtime resident of the Mount, and a woman whom Penny had cared for at home as a private duty aide. I've learned that people in nursing homes have innumerable euphemisms for the word "death." Penny said of Bob, "He went away." He was one of her favorites. "He dreamed of buying a boat—everyone would be invited to go," she said. "When you get to know your residents, they are like family." Penny herself was alone in Seattle. Most of her family remained in the Philippines; her only son was in the navy. "You get a bond with the residents. It's hard. Accepting death, before, it was hard for me to understand. The sisters [nuns] gave an in-service on death and dying. We have a lot of support, and that's helped a lot."

Bob's memorial service was held in the lovely chapel in the Mount, and staff and residents alike attended. "They can feel it's sad to lose someone," Penny said of the residents, many of whom have dementia.

This was my second visit to the Mount in two years, and the second time I had interviewed Penny. When we last spoke, she had told me how much she enjoyed joking with the residents. "One resident told me, 'You're a nut,'" she had said. "Another time I started singing to the radio, and a resident said, 'Don't quit your day job.'"

This time, she said she felt appreciated by the residents, their families, and Charlene Boyd, the dynamic administrator who is a national leader of the Pioneer Network. "This place—it's great to work," Penny said. "Anybody that leaves here—they want to come back. I see people working here twenty-five, thirty years. I'm going to retire here and find me a room!"

A call light came on, interrupting our conversation. She walked down the hall, knocked softly on the door, and said cheerfully, "Hi, Naomi." As I waited, a man came slowly by me in his wheelchair. He pushed the chair with his one good hand. "Slow way to China," he told me with a grin.

Penny passed by with a cup in her hand. The resident had drifted back to sleep, and her coffee had grown cold. Penny brought her a hot cup, again knocking on the door before entering.

Later, I interviewed Hipp Tiniacos, another aide who had worked in several nursing homes around the country. Like Penny, Hipp is an immigrant. He is from Greece, part of the Mount's little "United Nations," as one person described it. Hipp spoke with a deep sense of mission about his work. "What I like is the compassion—you have to take care of the residents. You are there for them. It's dedication to them. It's coming from inside of you, the love you can have about life, about people, they need that. They are looking for that."

The Mount, he agreed, was different from other places he had worked. "For the philosophy, the friendship, you always have answers when you need it. You never feel lost. The people you work with have a good heart to take care of the residents. They are very unique for that—they make you feel this is your home. They don't pressure you. Then that makes the residents feel home. Everybody works like a family."

He added that the door to Charlene's office was literally always open. At other facilities, the administration separated itself, physically and by attitude, from the life of the home. Here, he said, the office and nursing staff, the residents, and the families were all part of one community.

Marie McWalter, a longtime resident and a former nurse, seemed contented with her life at the Mount. "They want to make this as natural as possible, so they don't make too many rules or restrictions," she said. "I think they do an incredibly good job. The casualness with which they operate is part of the secret. For example, Charlene always calls you by name. She's an outstanding woman."

Further, Marie continued, "the people who are the cleaning people are just as respected as the others. It's as if there's no class distinction. You're treated as a person, with respect. We have meetings in which you can give your opinion. Some are very vocal, some are afraid to speak up."

Reflecting on her own nursing career, Marie said, "Professionalism is how you feel about yourself and how you treat others. Treat others as you would wish to be treated. I didn't believe in being standoffish to patients. I would put my arms around them and be human to them."

Penny, Hipp, and Marie represent the heart of relationship in a nursing home, that of the direct caregiver and the resident. As we have seen, aides, more than anyone else, determine whether a resident's day is good or bad. Without that strong relationship, the quality of life suffers. From that special place, relationships lead outward, connecting the residents to each other, to other staff throughout the nursing home, and to family members, both their own and others'.

Brenda Jennings has worked at the Mount since 1980, first as an aide and now as a registered nurse and neighborhood coordinator. Asked how life changed after the Mount switched to resident-directed care, she said, "There is a lot more caring connection between residents and staff. One resident volunteers to help with English classes with the staff. Another reads in another neighborhood to someone with multiple sclerosis. Another resident wrote a card for the staff. It's like an extended family."

Relationships spill over to life outside the walls of the nursing home. One nurse invited assisted-living residents to her wedding, and ten came. "They brought us gifts. We're not supposed to accept gifts, but the reality of the relationships I had with them made it impossible for me to refuse," she said.

The more time I spent in such places, the more I learned that culture change is fundamentally about relationships and community. Even with all the choices in the world, people would not be happy living in a nursing home if they lacked true companionship.

"Who *wouldn't* say that relationships are the most important thing in their life? Wouldn't you?" retorted assisted-living director and registered nurse Jana Brumbaugh with some exasperation, when I asked a group of nurse leaders at the Mount if relationships were key to a high quality of life in long-term care. "Wouldn't *you* say your family and your friends matter more than anything else?"

If anything, relationships are more important inside nursing homes than elsewhere. As many as 50 percent of residents are alone in the world; the family members of many others live far away. As one study put it, nursing homes have "an environment inherently torn between being a business and being a family for the residents."[1] Residents and their families hope and may even expect that the nursing home will become an extended family, where the individual will be appreciated for her unique experiences, pleasures, interests, and humor. Whether the employees can deliver on those expectations depends on how intentionally their leaders go about creating a community of warmth and compassion. If administrators demonstrate an uncaring attitude by not learning residents' names or, worse, by allowing poor treatment, the social support system quickly breaks down. If, like Charlene Boyd and Steve Shields, administrators demonstrate in clear and visible ways their commitment to relationships, they create an environment that fosters caring.

Garth Brokaw related one of his favorite images of life at Fairport Baptist: A resident held a young aide in his arms as they danced in the hall. I told him of Steve Shields's mother, who was rebuked by the nursing home for dancing in the hall. Garth shook his head. "Here," he said, "you can dance alone, or we'll dance with you."

A strong sense of community provides not only important social support, engagement, joy, and companionship, but also mutual respect and affection. Without this strong foundation, the basic clinical care may be wanting. Nursing homes without a sense of community and purpose are unlikely to retain aides or nurses (as we saw in Chapter 4). Turnover will perpetuate, short staffing will persist, and aides will insist they have no time to properly feed and bathe people, let alone sit around and reminisce with them.

The importance of relationships in long-term care is not news. In 1966, Herbert Shore, the granddaddy of nursing home transformation, wrote a stirring article called "New Ideas in Institutional Care." More than forty years later, his ideas are still fresh. Shore imagined a holistic community of elders whose physical, spiritual, emotional, and social needs were met. Citing a 1923 work by W. I. Thomas, he identified these simple human needs: "the need for security, . . . for new experience, . . . for affection, . . . for recognition."[2] Each of these assumes the need to be in community with others.

Those who embark on the mission of deep systemic change for nursing homes begin by discovering what residents most want and then trying to deliver it. As it turns out, what most frail elderly people want is no different from what the rest of us want from life: dignity, respect, freedom to make decisions, and—perhaps most of all—warm, loving relationships.[3] From that firm basis flows everything else: not only good physical care but also an end to Bill Thomas's three plagues of loneliness, helplessness, and boredom.

Yet the recognition of the value of relationship has been slow to penetrate the walls of many nursing homes. A friend asked me to join her on a visit to her mother, who was in the rehabilitation wing of a well-respected retirement community in the Washington, D. C., area. As soon as we entered, we saw what my friend said was typical: a coterie of white-coated staff looking bored and making small talk with each other, standing around the nurse's station. The patients, there to recover from injury or illness, were for the most part alone, other than one who was being walked down the hall with a physical therapist—an agency employee and not on staff. My friend's mother went on to recover. But what she perceived as uncaring attitudes of staff made her recovery more difficult.

"They put all their money into the plant and much less into staff training," my friend believed. "My mother waited for one hour for pain medication. The nurse said, 'I forgot.' Why couldn't it be that the staff and the patients take an interest in each other? Why can't they see the patients as real people with pasts they would want to get to know?"

Noting the high levels of loneliness among nursing home residents, an article in the *Journal of Gerontological Nursing* identifies the causes as the lack of intimate relationships, increased dependency, and loss of friends, home, independence, and self-identity.[4]

Some independent and assisted-living settings may not be any better in this regard. A study in the journal *Aging and Mental Health* found that loneliness and resulting depression often went unrecognized and untreated in two retirement facilities. Of 159 people in the study, 43—more than one-fourth—scored at the highest level on a loneliness scale and were at higher risk for depression. Although the idea of maintaining independence and control is a worthy one, often people in assisted living spend most of their time alone, emerging only for meals at assigned tables or the occasional group activity, but little else. A survey by social worker Sherry Cummings of residents in an assisted-living facility found their psychological well-being was closely related to the amount of social support they received. Moreover simply offering social programs was not enough, according to this researcher. She suggested assisted-living facilities develop strategies to enhance relationships among residents themselves and between residents and staff.[5]

An assisted-living center in my neighborhood had dozens of elders lined up, staring at soap operas on the obligatory big-screen television. The "apartments" were no more than private bedrooms and baths, lacking even a microwave oven or small refrigerator. The atmosphere was lifeless, with little interaction or engagement by the staff. Indeed, some people in assisted living, in an effort to fend off being moved to a nursing home, shun interactions with others for fear of revealing their frailties or forgetfulness.

Rx: Friendship

A growing body of research shows how critical the role of social support is to health and well-being for people of all ages. Researchers have conducted hundreds of studies on the relationships between physical health and friendship, loneliness, and social networks. Researcher Janice Kiecolt-Glaser of Ohio State University called the connection between satisfying personal relationships and better immune function "one of the most robust findings" in psychoneuroimmunology, which is the study of the biological mechanisms by which emotions, stress, and behavior affect resistance to disease.[6]

Much of this research flows from our growing understanding of the toll that stress takes on the body. The American Institute of Stress points out the serious health consequences of loneliness, social isolation, and feelings of worthlessness. Such insidious causes of stress contribute to a host of disorders, including heart attacks, asthma, diabetes, herpes, headaches, some types of cancer, even the common cold. In contrast, social support seems to have a buffering or protective effect. In a study of 169 centenarians, the only shared personality trait was the ability to manage stress well.[7]

Others studies have shown an association between social engagement and lower disability and mortality.

Clinical psychologist Joan Klagsbrun believes that "the next revolution of health care has to bring our attention to the health potential of both helping others and being supported by others." As a therapist, she pays attention to her clients' social networks and circle of friends.

According to Klagsbrun, strong relationships should be nurtured so that people feel they have true friends with whom they can be honest, not just a group with whom they have superficial, polite interactions. "Good support can make us feel cared for and worthy of love. Feeling embedded in the network or having a secure place has a profound effect on how we think and feel about our surroundings and ourselves and whether we feel affirmed and valuable," Klagsbrun told me in an interview. With older people, in particular, she recommends that caregivers practice what she calls "deep listening." "When elders' words are taken in and said back slowly to them—even fragments that might not make perfect sense—some meanings can emerge. When they feel regularly attended to in this manner, it can be empowering and even health-giving."

In numerous studies, people identify close relationships as the bread of life, without which there would be little point in waking up to a new day. People in nursing homes are no different. Twenty years ago, the National Citizens' Coalition for Nursing Home Reform conducted a study of four hundred residents in seventy nursing homes across the nation. Asked to identify what made for a high quality of life in a nursing home, residents most frequently mentioned having staff with good attitudes and feelings toward residents. Second on their list was a homelike atmosphere, and third was food. Further down were things like activities, medical care, and cleanliness.

Since then, many studies have examined the role of social support and quality of life in nursing homes. In four studies of older people who moved either from the community to a nursing home or from a state mental hospital to long-term care, researchers Morton Lieberman and Sheldon Tobin found that the psychosocial environment was a bigger factor in how people fared than were their psychological attributes. Topping the list was the "warmth expressed in interpersonal relations between residents and staff."[8]

In a survey about quality of life inside five long-term care sites, residents said what they missed most were such simple activities as "being able to bake cakes and entertain friends," "going food shopping with a friend," "belonging to an organization and going to meetings," and "having my car and going on Vegas trips." In the same survey, a far higher percentage of residents ranked contact with family and friends as very important to them than ranked physical problems as very important. In fact, a majority said physical problems were "not important" to their quality of life. This contrasted with the staff, of whom 85 percent ranked physical health as very important to residents' quality of life. And as much as redesigning the institution into a home is valued, residents in this study tended to believe that "care matters more than physical environment."[9]

Volunteers in a pet program that a nursing home piloted were surprised to learn their concerns about invading residents' privacy were often unfounded. Far more important to residents was the opportunity to chat, even with a stranger. "As institutionalized people, older women and men were often more concerned with getting personal attention than with preserving privacy," the researcher noted. One volunteer referred to the relationships formed during this time as "an unexpected intimacy."[10]

The longing for a caring community within the nursing home is also strong among the staff, according to many studies. When aides believe their employer values neither the residents nor supportive relationships, they are more likely to suffer stress and burnout on the job. In what he calls a "remarkable finding," Bill Thomas writes that "recent surveys of people who work with elders have found that the number one reason people stay in the field is the opportunity to create and sustain meaningful relationships with elders."[11] Staff who develop good relationships with residents report greater job satisfaction, which leads to reduced turnover rates.

It is discouraging, then, to learn that many nurses—who are leaders in any long-term care facility—may unintentionally behave in ways that prevent close relationships with those in their care. There is a disconnect between what some nurses perceive as providing good care and what patients or nursing home residents perceive as receiving good care. "Caring," according to a lengthy review in the nursing literature, means more than "a benevolent, technically competent, one-way care-provider interaction. Rather, the essential characteristic of caring is being with the proactive recipient of the care *who is more than an object to which the care-providers do things*" (emphasis added).[12] In one of the studies the review cited, which compared nurses' and nursing home residents' views on what "caring" meant, residents ranked "puts patient first no matter what else happens" as the most important caring behavior; nurses did not even include this behavior in their top ten. In other studies included in the literature review, residents generally put honest, open communication on a much higher plane than did nurses, whose "intent is more often about control rather than benevolence and another's best interests."

Other studies found that only the housekeeping staff took time to have normal conversations with residents.[13] Housekeepers, in fact, are an overlooked source of companionship to people in both long-term care and hospitals.

In yet another study, nurses who work in nursing homes were urged to assess residents' loneliness and conduct "interventions," such as "actively participate in conversations with the resident," "spend time with the resident during routine care," and "assist the resident to make phone calls and write letters."[14]

What does it say about nursing homes that a respected nursing journal considers such advice worth publishing? Is it not troubling that the notion of having a conversation with someone you see every day is not taken for granted but described as an "intervention"?

Particularly appalling was an article in the *Journal of Nursing Scholarship* that questioned whether "a meaningful provider-resident relationship is a realistic outcome in long-term care environments." While acknowledging that gerontological nursing experts believe close relationships should be "the hallmark of good geriatric nursing care," the researchers were skeptical that such a goal is achievable.[15]

Again, it is not that nurses are callous. As one nurse attending a culture-change workshop told me: "People [working in long-term care] *do* care. Why else would we stay?" The system, however, drives nurses to focus not on relationships but on enforcing regulations, holding to strict medication regimes, and running a tight ship.

In contrast, the nurses I encountered in transformative homes demonstrated that meaningful relationships not only were possible but improved the quality of their work. In every home I visited, I encountered wonderful nurses who were energized by being part of a team of compassionate caregivers. Without their knowledge, skills, and willingness to share power, culture change would not be possible.

At Pleasant View in New Hampshire, when the administration was beginning its efforts to change the culture, the residents' community council made it clear that developing strong relationships with staff was primary to them. One of the council's first and most significant demands was that the administration stop hiring agency workers. "Our residents didn't like agency staff—someone different every day who didn't know what they liked or needed. They were constantly having to explain to each new person. That was their first loud comment. We asked how could we make it better? They said, if we each had our own staff," said Barbara Platts-Comeau, who headed Pleasant View's culture-change team.

As Pleasant View's community councils grew, residents became more confident and vocal. They began to write letters to the staff, which Barbara copied and put with the appropriate employees' paychecks. The first letter was full of criticisms of the care they received. "At first staff were angry," said Barbara. "But we said, 'Wait a minute. This is their home. We are guests in their home.'"

One active resident was Ruth, a lively woman full of fun, who wore a lavender muumuu and sporty glasses with red frames. She had lived at Pleasant View for two years. She could no longer walk, and her knees were very bad. "I had a big adjustment to make," she said. "I did my share of crying. But I adjusted. I'm doing fine now."

She enjoyed attending meetings of the community council and of the committee set up to implement culture change. Although the committee's goal was to make the place more homelike, Ruth said, "It's not exactly like your home, but it's comfortable. You can have your possessions that mean something to you." She was pleased that her suggestion to get two whirlpool tubs in good operating order was acted upon.

Wesley Village in Connecticut took the principles developed by Planetree for patient-centered care in hospitals and adapted them to its nursing home, creating what it calls the "relationship-centered approach to continuing care" (see Appendix D). "We looked at the research that had been done on elderly people living with chronic diseases," said the young and energetic administrator Heidi Gil. "The research on what impacts quality of life is vast and compelling. It really emphasizes the importance of community, faith, and relationships. It's about building a community with strong relationships and personal growth, no matter what age you are."

Everyone on the staff, in all departments, as well as volunteers, is encouraged and expected to be part of the tight-knit community. For example, Jordan Cohen, a housekeeper, knew several residents had old phonograph records that they cherished, but no way to play them. "The community has many CD and tape players but not a record player," explained Heidi. "Jordan took the initiative to bring in his own record player so that the residents could listen to the records." They enjoyed it so much that he later went out on his own to purchase a record player. This inspired all the housekeepers to contribute to the purchase. The housekeeping staff surprised the residents with the record player as a Christmas gift. In another instance, a dietary aide learned that a resident shared her love of limericks. The aide's grandmother had read her limericks and she had a treasured limerick book, which she gave to the resident.

"We form relationships with residents," said Joselma Cousens, a dietary aide. "We spend a lot of time with them. If we notice a problem, we tell someone and they listen to us."

As one way to strengthen relationships at Wesley Village, twenty-five volunteers, many of them staff members, collect stories of residents. The stories help distinguish each resident as an individual. The "Vital Life Stories" collection is kept in thick binders and open to staff, volunteers, and family members. When I visited Wesley Village, Julie Norko, a public relations staff member, had volunteered her time to collect stories. Resident Joyce Walsh, eighty-three, said, "At first I didn't think I had a story." But Julie prompted her to share childhood memories. Joyce reviewed and approved the final product before it was made available to others to read.

"My father always had a big garden," Joyce told me. She and her brothers and sisters helped plant and weed. The family grew enough potatoes to last through the winter. "My mother put up a hundred quarts of tomatoes," she said.

One of her parents' rules was that no one could go to bed angry at another family member. She recalled once being punished and sent to bed without supper. "An hour later, my mother was sneaking up, bringing me food," she said, laughing.

Julie had been collecting such stories from residents for two years. "I get so much out of it, to make these connections," she said. "Now I'm friends with Joyce. I'm getting her canning expertise."

The strands of culture change—honoring choice, empowering staff, making a homey environment—come together to create community. Sherry Smith, a young aide from Meadowlark Hills, admitted she thought the whole idea of having households with permanent assignments was "ridiculous." Convinced it would never work, she resigned as the change got under way. When she returned to visit, though, she realized how much better life had become for residents. She asked if she could come back and now works in a household there. "I think it's the best thing we've ever done," she said, her eyes filling with tears. "It's not too many people who can say they love coming to work every day."

I was surprised by how often staff members were moved to tears as they talked to me about their work.

"People cry a lot around here," I told Steve Shields. He laughed and told me, "I always say if you haven't had a good hard cry in front of everybody, then you haven't changed anything."

At Meadowlark, I attended a learning circle, a method used by several transformative homes—and many other organizations as well—to give everyone a voice. Staff and residents use learning circles to defuse problems, foster connectedness, and create a safe space for those who are shy or who have trouble speaking. Everyone is given a chance to talk about a given theme—from a favorite holiday memory to complaints about the food. For those who physically can't speak, there are learning circles that engage their other senses by passing around objects that are pleasing to the touch or smell.

At one learning circle I attended, the group shared with me how they experienced life at Meadowlark.

"It's all about the relationships of the staff—they are so loving and caring," said one woman. "We aren't kept dependent."

Another disagreed. She had recently waited a long time for someone to respond to her call light. She thought the care could be improved.

A third woman reflected on how she felt upon returning to Meadow-lark after being in the hospital for surgery. "I couldn't believe that when I returned, three people came in and said how happy they were to see me and how much they missed me. I like it here so much. My daughter was so surprised when I said I don't know if I'd even want to return home."

As the second woman indicated, life is not perfect, no matter how many strides have been made. At almost every home I visited, there were residents whose call light had not been answered promptly, or who had gone through a bad experience with an aide or with another resident, or who was sick of the food or feeling low. Nursing homes are human enterprises filled with people with complex problems, so there will always be mistakes and sorrow. Residents bring their own dispositions that they have had for a lifetime—spunky or shy, grumpy or wisecracking. As one daughter said to me of her mother, who lived at the Mount, "My mother complains a lot. But she always complained a lot."

The goal cannot be a complaint-free place, but rather a place where complaints can be honestly shared and handled. Is the environment one of hope, of compassion, of humor, of "normalcy"? Some people even argue that spending your last years in a caring community can be preferable to staying in your own home.

A woman who had recently moved to an assisted-living apartment at the Mount said: "I moved in anticipation that I may need more help in the future. I wanted to be in a place, if something developed. The earlier people move in, the better they adjust."

Another woman chimed in, saying that before she moved there, "I had two friends left. I figured if I came here, there'd be more than two people at my funeral!"

I often heard this sentiment expressed. Rather than wait for a crisis or for the time they are "too far gone" to be appreciated for the person they have always been, some choose to move when they can still easily form friendships.

Bill Thomas takes it a step further. In his call to arms, *What are Old People For?* he proclaims: "We must overcome outmoded and dysfunctional ideas about independence and the hallowed role of the private home, which, no matter how lonely, isolated and boring, is deemed to be the *only* acceptable place to live" (emphasis his).[16]

In fact, said LaVrene Norton, "A nursing home is the ideal place to create community." But too many operators fail to grasp what this means. "I once had a nursing home client who wanted McDonald's to be the model for the industry," LaVrene said. In a similar vein, the nation's first assisted-living administration program, at George Mason University, collaborates with Disney to learn about hospitality and customer relations.

So what's wrong with that? Certainly the intentions behind such efforts are not bad: treating people who live in long-term care as valued customers is certainly better than treating them as nobodies to be pushed around. But the answer to what elders need does not appear in a corporate franchise manual. What people need in their day-to-day lives is a genuine community based on mutual respect, affection, and the deep intimacy that comes with being present for people who have faced profound loss and who seek to find both meaning and pleasure in their remaining years.

"It's all about the journey. There is no destination," said Bill Thomas. "The pursuit for well-being in community will go on as long as there are human communities. It's not a 'customer service.' It's not built around hospitality, but dignity, love, and affection. When elders can live a life rich in those virtues, we repair the world, and we build a better life for people of all ages."

> We envision for our Residents normalcy and individualized, quality care. We will work in partnership to create the best of "home": an environment of friendship, spontaneity, creativity, comfort and pleasure. We envision a place where each of us is known; where each is comfortable being one's self, where each of us wants to be. And, we envision a thriving and growing community, full of life and vitality, in which all are welcome and all contribute.
>
> —Vision statement developed by nursing home staff at
> Fairport Baptist Homes, Rochester, New York

> Remember the moments of the past
> Look forward to the promise of the future
> But most of all: celebrate
> The present for it is precious.
>
> —From a bulletin board at the Mount

Chapter 7

From the Top of the Ferris Wheel
Breaking Barriers

> We would drive her here and there, just to get her out of there. It's so difficult to break people out. She had severe osteoporosis so she could barely move, but she wanted to get out. She counted on one sister coming to get her once a week, and me once a month. It would exhaust her, but she lived for it.
>
> —Gay Hanna, on her mother's nursing home experience

"I forgot how big the sky is"

My friend Lynne's aunt had lived in a nursing home for only a few months. But her world had rapidly shrunk. The cloistered institution had already clouded her memory of the wide Kansas sky she had known all her life. On her first outing, she looked around in amazement.

Lynne cried when she told me this story. Her aunt's comment captured all the painful loss that accompanies life in a nursing home. Later I would visit the place where Lynne's mother and aunt lived—the typical one-story brick building in a small town. The room Lynne's mother shared with a stranger was impossibly tiny, with enough space only for two narrow beds and bureaus. Although it was a sunny summer afternoon, the building seemed dark and too quiet. The one note of levity, a 1950s-style ice cream parlor, only accented the sad surroundings. The staff was kind to her mother and aunt, Lynne said, but there was little to keep residents engaged, happy—or able to remember how big the sky is.

The scene not far away at Crestview, in rural Missouri, could not have been more different. There, under the leadership of Eric and Margie Haider, staff members broke through the customary barriers between those living inside a nursing home and the outside world. "Ninety-five percent of nursing homes assume that if you're ninety, you're going to love to play bingo for a banana," said Eric. "Maybe I want to play bingo for five hundred dollars at a bingo parlor. Take me there! Take me to a casino! What crime have they done that they've lost this privilege? We ask them what they want to do."

The staff I interviewed at Crestview were enthusiastic, even volunteering to accompany residents on outings after work hours. Eric said that he had a waiting list of eighty potential employees, thanks to word of mouth. When aides at other homes hear that their counterparts at Crestview get paid to go fishing with residents, he said, they too want to work there. "My employees are my best advertisement," he said. Most Crestview employees had driver's licenses and were encouraged to take residents out. Crestview paid a small extra insurance premium to cover them.

Charlie, a tall, lanky guy with a hangdog expression and drooping mustache, was a prime instigator. One of his favorite stories was of the time he invited residents to go to the Harrison County fair. He went three times, taking as many people as he could.

One evening, when they got to the rides, some wanted to go on the merry-go-round. "One little lady, I got her on the Ferris wheel, and they stopped us up on top," Charlie recalled. "I said, 'Elsie, I was doing pretty good until they did this.' She said, 'Yeah.' I said, 'Elsie, how long's it been since you been on a Ferris wheel?' She said, 'Charlie, I ain't never been on a Ferris wheel.' She was a hundred years old."

I love the image of Charlie and hundred-year-old Elsie stuck on top of the Ferris wheel, the seat swinging lightly as they gaze out over the midway. The scene is so life affirming, joyful, spontaneous. Elsie challenges every notion we have about who lives in nursing homes.

The staff insisted that many residents were eager for adventure, even as their families were convinced their loved ones were "too far gone." Even those on the "heavy care unit"—those who were the most debilitated—enjoyed getting out. One aide on the unit invited residents to go out on a lake on her brother's pontoon boat. "Well, you don't have any trouble finding volunteers—if you say you're going to do something like that, these people will jump," Charlie said. "We went two times. That's twenty-seven miles away. We took them fishing. We had fifty-six residents at the lake and twenty-nine staff members. They always want to do a fish fry afterwards. The secret to this is, you include housekeepers, laundry, and kitchen."

At Meadowlark Hills, Steve Shields tells a story that he says has become legend. It all began when Sarah, an aide in one of the households, asked "Hannah," a resident, what she would like to do that evening. After giving the matter some thought, Hannah said, "I'd like to rent a limousine and go dancing."

Sarah said, "Well, okay, do you want to go by yourself or get some others?"

Hannah said she'd like to get others to join her, so she got her walker and went to three households in Meadowlark, asking who wanted to rent a limo and go dancing. She soon recruited a carful of six adventurous residents.

That evening, "a big white limo pulled up, and they loaded it full of hardware—there's wheelchairs, walkers, four-pronged canes—it was like a modern art sculpture," said Steve. They chose to go to a country-and-western dive that Steve describes as "the biggest redneck bar in Manhattan." When Hannah crossed the threshold, she said, "Let's party!"

There were only four men slumped over the bar, and apparently they had never seen anything quite like this. They craned their necks to watch as the group order a few pitchers of beer. Steve went on:

> One can't stand it any longer. He gets up and walks over and says, 'What have we got going here?' One of the residents says, 'Well, we're partying, you want some beer?' He said, 'Well, all right.' He sits down with them, and the other three start coming over, and they all start drinking. Hannah asked one to dance, and they put on a two-step, and they all started dancing, and they really just party. It got kind of late—about 8:30—it was time to go. They'd all bonded, and so the guys helped them out to the car and got them all tucked in. Hannah opened the window and waves with her fingers and said, 'Bye, boys.' As they were pulling out, the lead guy slapped his knee and said, 'Well, goddamn, when I get old, I want to move to Meadowlark too.'

Steve explained how this story encapsulates the principles of the households they have created at Meadowlark.

> For one, a nurse's aide, or anybody else, would not ask the resident in a traditional model what they'd like to do tonight, because nobody even has an idea that is an option—that someone has a personal choice. Or else they're too busy to even ask. The second thing is that Hannah wasn't just musing. That's what she wanted to do, and she had no reason to think that she couldn't. The culture had been established enough they knew if they wanted to do something, they'd do it. The other thing is we make ghettos out of these places. It was so unusual that some human beings who happen to have some apparatus and a few wrinkles would go to a bar and have a drink and do the two-step. It confounded the [men in the

bar]. It didn't fit. You had to get up and ask what was going on. For those guys, it changed their sense of their whole future. Everyone has a feeling of denial or fear around this getting old and frail and put in a place. At least for that moment, it was a knee-slapper—he'll move to Meadowlark too! He's picturing he can still come down to the bar. On the face of it, it's a humorous story. But it's a very deep story.

Dreaming Big

P. K. Beville has been a psychologist in long-term care for more than twenty-five years. In that capacity, she has been called in to conduct assessments of people in long-term care who were having behavior problems. What she learned through this work transformed her thinking of who lives in nursing homes. "What I was finding, the behaviors were actually a function of trying to control their environment, rather than psychosis or anything like that," she said. "The beauty of what I saw was so stunning. There was such a dichotomy between the environment that they were in, which was very poor, and their human spirit, which was very positive. Nine times out of ten underneath that layer of resignation was a fun-loving person that you could get glimpses of."

She went on to found Second Wind Dreams, a nonprofit based in DeLand, Florida. Part Make-a-Wish Foundation, part *Queen for a Day*, Second Wind Dreams fulfills long-held desires of people in long-term care. On the organization's website are photos of older people doing all sorts of things, from riding a camel to conducting an orchestra, straddling a Harley, receiving an honorary college degree, or simply connecting with long-lost relatives. Beville says the results of her work go far beyond the momentary thrill each elder experiences. "People treat it like fluff, but the changes are far deeper than the actual dream," she said. She conducted a study of people in three nursing homes who were participating in Second Wind Dreams. Using the Geriatric Depression Scale, a basic screening tool, she measured depression in residents before and after the Second Wind Dreams program was in place. Ten months after the program began, depression overall among residents was down by 56 percent, staff morale had increased by 62 percent, and staff turnover had dropped by 8 percent, changes Beville attributes to her program, although the study was not controlled for other variables.

Beville also sees Second Wind Dreams as a way to bridge the divide between the wider community and the nursing home. Increasingly, she implements the program with outside volunteers. "I'm learning the community is reaching out to the nursing home," she said. "I think that will create the culture change. We're learning the volunteers are ready to take the cutting edge on this thing. High school students, Rotary Clubs, individuals are all adopting nursing homes. It's just been an amazing outpouring, once we realized the focus needs to be on the volunteers, who will then be the catalyst for the dreams to come true." Beville hopes her program will change public perceptions of what it means to be old and disabled.

The chance for nursing home residents to partake in normal life—whether by getting out of the home or engaging with people who don't live or work there—adds seasoning and spark to what might otherwise be a dull routine. At Teresian House in Albany, New York, an energetic staff member, Colleen Fowler, who had worked her way up from dietary aide and was training to be a licensed practical nurse, told me her "brainstorm" was taking a group to the races at Saratoga. Fourteen nursing home residents piled into the Teresian House bus, with staff members following along in cars. "We take them out to the community—to the theater, on fishing trips," she said. "One resident had a nephew who was a park officer, and he got us in for free to Grafton Lakes State Park."

Trips to such ordinary places as restaurants, shopping malls, fishing holes, and picnic groves—outings that most of us take for granted— are rare treats to most residents of nursing homes, who must depend on others to transport and escort them.

Garth Brokaw described how culture change at Fairport Baptist led his staff to broaden their view of who could leave the nursing home.

One of the big changes around here was we always had what was called Dutch treats, where we take a group out to a restaurant. The procedure was that therapeutic recreation staff would go through and talk to Nursing and they'd say, 'Well, Mrs. Jones, she can go, she's appropriate, and Mr. Harvey, we better leave him back, because he drools. So he's not appropriate.' Once we got into this model, the staff came to us and said, 'If we're going out to a restaurant, we're all going.' So now they're all going, and that includes all the staff.

We've got a couple restaurants here in Rochester that I guess will never be the same—but everybody goes. People who are on a puree diet, the staff sit down and figure out what's on that menu that they can handle. Or they will take something—a slurry—to break down food so that it's easier to swallow. Staff becomes very creative when you allow it and encourage it.

Segregation within Continuing-Care Retirement Communities

Paradoxically, retirement communities—even those claiming to offer the very best in full-service living—can be as guilty as the rest of us when it comes to shunting nursing home residents off to the side. Continuing-care retirement communities, or CCRCs, promise older people the opportunity to "age in place" through a lifelong continuum of care. Many CCRCs are considered the top-of-the-line option in eldercare in their communities, and some will not accept Medicaid payments.

Generally, you move into your own apartment or townhouse in a CCRC as an independent person. Then, if your needs increase, you move to either assisted living or the nursing home on campus. The cost to move to a CCRC is substantial—from at least $100,000 to as high as $500,000, depending on location and size of the dwelling—in addition to monthly service fees for rent and one or more meals a day. In 2006, 600,000 Americans lived in 2,240 CCRCs.[1] You pay, in part, for the security of knowing that no matter how ill—or broke—you become, the community will continue to care for you. Many older people find comfort in the idea that they will never be a burden on their children. They enjoy the community of peers and a rich social and educational calendar of lectures, cultural performances, and field trips.

But CCRCs' promise of aging in place sometimes doesn't work out the way people imagine. Yes, you can stay on the campus, but leaving your independent apartment for long-term care often disrupts your social ties. There is a strong stigma in many continuing-care retirement communities attached to those who need more help. Thus, even as people pay for the security of lifelong care, they are in denial—or perhaps simple fear—that they will ever need that care. Retirement communities often reinforce this denial through de facto segregation of nursing home residents. The official campus tour, for example, may avoid the nursing home and assisted-living areas.

According to Sheryl Zimmerman, a noted long-term care researcher with the University of North Carolina: "One of the beauties of a CCRC is people really can age in place within that one community. But in some cases, there's a certain fallacy related to that. You're still moving from your independent apartment to assisted living or to the nursing home. We know from the research, people do feel that really is moving, although there is a familiarity with the other people who live there, sometimes. The other thing we've heard is there's a lot of stigma. We're concerned that people who could benefit from the care, where there are more services they actually need, people aren't wanting to go there."

Some CCRCs have a culture that encourages independent residents to spend time with people who live in assisted living or the nursing home. But many others do not. At a faith-based continuing-care retirement community I visited in the Midwest, a staff member, "Jane," pulled me aside. Part of her job was to coordinate Guest Night. This was a regular event for both current and prospective residents of the retirement community. It included a special dinner and a stimulating program. Jane, who had worked at this CCRC for ten years, had always included nursing home residents who wished to attend the event. But two years earlier, management had instructed her to stop including them. Why? Because the dinner was not really a social event for the community but a marketing tool. Potential customers might not want to move there if they pictured rubbing elbows with "those people"—those in wheelchairs, those who repeat themselves, those whose hearing or vision is fading, those who have trouble eating. "I fought hard and used every argument I could think of, but I lost," Jane said sadly. Management "compromised" by allowing individual nursing home residents to attend if they received a specific invitation from an independent resident—effectively ending their inclusion. The policy was especially painful for Jane when her own mother had to move from the independent section to the nursing home. Her mother had particularly enjoyed the guest nights. Jane eventually started a pizza and movie night for the nursing home, but it was not the same.

Management's policies merely reflected a prevalent attitude. Other elders in CCRCs, still capable, often avoid those who have "lost it." Some may feel awkward and not know how to communicate with a person with dementia, for example. After all, it's not easy. Others may find it too painful to see dear friends no longer able to communicate or to remember them. But some shun all contact with nursing home residents, no matter what their ailment.

John Erickson, CEO of Erickson Retirement Communities, acknowledges the problem. He believes that seeing someone in decline is a frightening reminder to healthier elders of what may lie in store for them. He told me of a group of four men in one of his communities who were great friends. They ate dinner together every night, taking turns bringing a bottle of wine. Eventually, one of them developed medical problems and had to move to the nursing home building. After he had settled in, Erickson paid him a visit to find out how he was getting along.

"Not so good," the man told him. "You know, I ate dinner with those guys for two years, and I've now been here four months and not one of them has come to see me."

A friend whose father lives in a CCRC shared a similar tale. When his father was doing poorly and thought he might need more help, he wanted to leave the CCRC. "I believe [the nursing home] is pretty stigmatized there," my friend said. "I think that folks feel that when you check in at assisted care, the show's over. My dad didn't want to be thought of as 'one of them.' He's even queasy about visiting people that have been shipped over there—people he knows! I don't judge him. I know it must be hard to be in his shoes."

Ironically, although culture-change leaders want to break down these barriers, in one home it was the resident-choice philosophy that had the opposite effect. At the Methodist Home in Washington, D.C., Mary Savoy, director of health services, explained how they were changing the dining experience to accommodate residents' wishes. In this case, residents who still functioned well wanted to eat separately from those who needed more assistance. The home honored this request by sectioning off a part of the dining room with potted plants to create a more private area for those without visible problems.

I asked her if she was concerned about what would happen when someone began to fail and would have to cross over to the other side of the potted plants. In fact, she said, it already was happening with one woman. "That resident and the relationships she's formed with the folks that she eats with is very much in consideration. We're reaching the time where she won't be able to eat with them. I don't know what's going to happen. We decided not to move her just yet. But we have to figure the dining experience from her experience and the folks she eats with. If we can get a family member to sit with her at mealtime, that might be a distraction for her and she could stay. But it is complex."

Complex indeed. How is a nursing home or any congregate setting supposed to juggle such ethical questions as the rights or interests of the individual versus the group? Ideally, in a place such as the Green House or any household of elders, there will be enough tolerance and affection that each individual's declining abilities will be accepted. Working toward that ideal seems to be what the journey of transformation is all about. But there are no simple answers.

That is what made a comment by an independent resident of Traceway in Tupelo all the more impressive. Bea McBryde said that in the past, she had dreaded the prospect of moving to Cedars, the traditional nursing home. Her daughter, a nurse, did not want her ever to have to go there. "The Cedars is too institutional for me. I'm sure you get good care, but there's nothing to look forward to," Bea said.

But she felt differently about the Green Houses. "The Green House is so pretty. And the shahbaz treats you so nice when you go down there. That's were I'm going when I leave here," she said happily. She was the only person I interviewed who seemed to welcome the prospect of moving to "the other side" of a CCRC. The Green House must be doing something right.

Bringing the Outside In

To fundamentally change an entrenched institutional culture takes strong leadership.

At the Mount, I met Juanita Webb, a resident of the nursing home, who had grown up in Seattle. She had raised three sons and worked as a parish secretary. She had been a widow for decades, having lost her husband to cancer when he was only forty. Over time, she grew tired of living alone. She had fond memories of the Mount, having sung carols there as a child. "There was no question where I would go," she said of her decision to move there.

When I met Mrs. Webb, she had endured many physical problems, from a knee replacement to double pneumonia. She was in considerable pain and eventually had to move from the Mount's assisted-living side to a nursing home household down the hall. Despite moving to "the other side," as residents referred to it, Mrs. Webb said: "I still go to meetings in assisted living. [Administrator] Charlene [Boyd] told me, 'You go on doing exactly what you've been doing.'" She deeply appreciated this support from Charlene, and she continued to participate in daily life throughout the Mount.

Without such intentional leadership in a community, separation and isolation will persist. Loneliness and lack of friendships affect our physical and mental well-being and contribute significantly to stress, no matter what our age or living situation (see Chapter 6).

Ideally, all aspects of a nursing home or assisted-living center reflect a sense of community, from the physical design of a place to its programs and relationships. At Evergreen in Oshkosh, for example, the main social area of the community, a café, is in the center of the nursing home.

At Kendal at Oberlin, the only access to the wood-and-glass swimming pavilion is through the nursing home. The campus was designed to be inclusive. "If you live in a cottage on the west side of our campus, you're going to go through our health center [nursing home] every day to get your mail and to come for your meals," said administrator Barbara Thomas. "It's to make sure our residents never become isolated in any level of care."

One resident, Ina, had embodied the openness of Kendal. She had ended up in the nursing home when she was only in her sixties, after a massive stroke left her partially paralyzed and with difficulty speaking. Kendal was not the first place she had moved. The first "was a beautiful facility," said her son, Gary Kornblith, "but it had very separate, independent living and nursing care areas. Mom was not welcome in the dining room, even if we took her."

At Kendal, though, she became integrated into the community. "People would sit down with her at dinner," said Kornblith. "She represented in a sense what was special about the Kendal philosophy, in that here was someone unable to do lots of things, but she was still fun to have around. We used to joke they needed a bar for her to hang out in."

His mother loved the jazz club on campus, and people began recommending CDs to her. She was known for her lifelong sense of fashion. Kornblith recalls:

> She said, "So I'm old and disabled—that doesn't mean I can't wear flashy clothes." People knew it was meant to radiate a certain joy and fun.
>
> Kendal was really wonderful for her. The folks there were eager to encourage her to be as independent as she could. Towards the end, there were new issues and problems, but what impressed me was how there was a collective sense of making everything work at each step. There were communication glitches, but Mom knew she was loved, and she loved back. It wasn't just me and the family, it was with the staff and the other residents. It was very special.

Transformational homes make strong efforts not only to get residents out into the community, but to bring the community into the nursing home or to break down the walls that divide residents from the outside world. A core component of the Eden Alternative, for example, includes children as a regular part of residents' everyday life.

Ask most nursing homes if residents have opportunities to interact with children, and you will be assured that they do. "Oh, yes, the Girl Scout troop comes every Christmas to sing carols" is a standard response. As enjoyable as such encounters might be, they are too infrequent and too brief to be meaningful.

Researchers have studied what makes intergenerational programs successful. They recommend having close, rather than casual, contact and predictable, scheduled visits. Activities should be mutually rewarding and cooperative, rather than only performances by the children. Meaningful relationships are based on friendship, not charity.

The Mount has an exemplary Intergenerational Learning Center. Some one hundred children come to the on-site day-care centers, Monday through Friday. Architect Dyke Turner designed the day-care centers so that anyone walking through the building can easily enjoy watching the children play. Some of the children's rooms have wide-open doorways, just steps from a nursing home neighborhood. As I strolled down the indoor Main Street, I often stopped to look through a large window at toddlers busy at play. The children would stop and smile or wave, then get back to business.

The lives of youngsters and elders were woven together. Turning a corner, I came across two gentlemen in wheelchairs with a small group of four-year-olds on the carpet at their feet, all of them engrossed in a storybook an aide was reading. Elders are invited to eat in the day-care centers, and children come regularly to a particular neighborhood and visit with residents. Children and residents can take art classes together every week. Outdoors, elders sit on benches and watch youngsters clamor around a large playground of wooden swings and jungle gyms.

According to Joan Whitley, director of the Intergenerational Learning Center, the residents are welcome to come to the day-care centers anytime they wish. "Some just adopt us and come frequently," she said. "They stay as long as they want and help us. Other people just meet kids throughout the building. Different things develop. A particular resident bonds with a child-care aide. They become good buddies. That friendship helps inform the kids."

Neighborhood coordinator Brenda Jennings told of an eighty-year-old man who was raised in an orphanage who had no grandchildren. "He loves to be around the kids and to hang out in the day-care center. One of the teachers asked if it would be okay to give him a surprise party. He glowed for weeks. I think being with kids is healing for him."

Unlike the Mount, the nursing home in my neighborhood discouraged my neighbor from bringing her baby to visit residents. Ellen had hoped to be a regular volunteer there, giving elders the chance to know her son, and him a chance to be around older people, since his grandparents live far away. Rather than welcome her, the nursing home refused her offer. Its policy was that all volunteers must have a TB test, and her baby had not had one. The elders who live there of course were not given the opportunity to weigh in on the issue.

Not that all residents enjoy having children around—some want nothing to do with them. When I was walking through the Mount with a nurse, we saw a small group of two-year-olds playing in a neighborhood. "I wish you nice ladies would take these things away," a resident said to us, pointing to the children. She may have lost the word "children," but she got her meaning across.

Maggie Lucas, who brought her two children to the day-care center at the Mount, said the sense of community there was important to her family. Her children's grandparents do not live nearby, so she appreciated having other elders involved in their lives. "We love the diversity of the population, both nationally and agewise. My kids don't blink an eye at respirators or wheelchairs or people with one leg. The children visit the same neighborhood in the nursing home every week. The kids know who has a dog that likes to be petted, who has a cat you should leave alone, who gives out candy," she said.

While I was visiting, a group of junior high students from a Catholic school made their monthly visit to one of the neighborhoods. They were going to decorate Valentine's Day cookies with ten or so residents, two of whom had been coaxed to join in by the recreation therapist. "I didn't want to come," said one. "I had taken my bath and was tired." When the coast was clear, she wheeled herself back to her room.

The other woman stayed and seemed to enjoy the activity in spite of herself. With her one good hand, she attempted to mix food coloring into white frosting. She laughed at the mess she felt she was making.

When the young teens arrived, they were full of enthusiasm. "I love coming," said one girl. "It's so fun here." The kids told me they had helped make a gingerbread house and paper snowflakes during past visits.

"Are you wearing eyeliner?" one girl asked her friend.

"These are intense cookies," another said.

The residents had stopped helping but were smiling, enjoying the students' conversation and watching them pour thick layers of sprinkles on the icing.

There are many wonderful stories of nursing home residents being part of real life. At the Mount, Mrs. Webb told me: "In the summer, there are tables outside. Every Friday night there's a jazz band. We can eat out there. People from the neighborhood come in. People dance rock and roll. It's good. It's loud and it's nice."

Lenawee Medical Care Facility in Michigan was the first in the nation to house a licensed Head Start center inside its nursing home. Olga, a staffer there, said, "I love seeing the way the residents come more alive when children come into the room. We went to a dining room, and a resident was dozing. A child touched him, and the smile on his face—I will never forget it. The kids love them and learn their names, and to see the young children respect their elders—there are a lot of pluses."

A teenage theater group uses Teresian House's theater for rehearsals and performances. Teresian House also has an on-site day-care center for children of staff, as does Fairport Baptist and Kendal at Oberlin.

Residents of an Apple Health Care home sponsored Little League teams. At the beginning of the season, the coach brought the kids to the nursing home to meet everyone. Residents went to the games and cheered on their team. At the season's end, residents hosted a celebration in the nursing home for the kids.

At Ridgewood in New Hampshire, culture-change leader Theresa Smith plans events every couple of months to celebrate the culture they are creating. She tries to think of ways to bridge generations and to make the nursing home a fun and inviting place for family members of both residents and staff. The first event was an "Evening under the Stars." Dozens of residents, staff, and family members gathered at dusk around a fire pit. During a learning circle, each person was asked to share a favorite summertime memory. A talking stick was passed around the circle, and whoever held the stick could share. One woman who never spoke talked. The group sang songs, roasted marshmallows, and made s'mores. Theresa said, "What was really touching was the stories that they told. And they talked about if for a long time after. It stayed with them."

Chapter 8

Beyond Bingo

Finding Meaning in Late Life

I do not think the remedy is in going to things or learning
to make mats. (Mrs. Henderson, who is in charge of all that,
came to see me yesterday and told me I could make really
pretty things, if I let her show me the way.) I also feel a great
heaviness at the thought of all these pressures to come—the
sight of the same Thanksgiving decoration, at the front door
as I passed it yesterday, opened a vista of years of it, years
of Santa Claus and the blind accordion player, while the
weariness of the flesh increases.

—Joyce Horner, *That Time of Year: A Chronicle
of Life in a Nursing Home*

At the risk of being trite, those thinking about long-term care
for older people must consider the meaning of life for life's
last decades. In actuality, long-term care discussions often
bog down in technicalities, which, though important, fail to
strike at the heart of the matter.

—Rosalie A. Kane, "Long-Term Care and a Good Quality
of Life"

I met Jean at the end of my visit to Pleasant View in Concord, New Hampshire. She was in bed, resting before dinner. She said she would ask me
to sit down, but—she waved her hand at the tiny half-room, where there was
no space for a chair.

Jean moved to the nursing home after having had three strokes and two
heart attacks. "But I'm a tough Yankee," she said. She appreciated the staff's

efforts to institute resident-directed care. Although she faced challenges there, she said, "I have a sense of humor, and I've kept it."

Her husband regularly came to see her and was now taking care of their household. "He's doing things I used to do—if I'd known he could do them, he would have done it long ago!" she said.

Jean quickly dispensed with my questions about her life in the nursing home. That was far less interesting than all that came before.

For the next hour, anecdotes of her life came pouring out. She was born here in Concord. She was "a good hard worker" who had held many jobs, the last one in a grocery store. She had four children, as well as grandchildren. One daughter was a phone engineer, and a son was a maintenance man. She was proud of them all. "I love my daughter-in-law, too—and my ex [daughter in law]," she said. "I don't get in their business." When the weather was nice, her family wheeled her around the grounds at Pleasant View, which seemed like a country manor.

She had been a quilter. Her quilts have been in many shows, and she especially enjoyed making baby quilts. She liked choosing fabric colors and prints. "Quilts are comforting," she said.

When she worked at the grocery, she learned how to decorate cakes. I observed that she must be very artistic, what with her quilting and cake decorating, and she nodded with pride. "Maybe I could be Grandma Moses," she said, only half-kidding.

On and on her stories came. Her niece in Tennessee sends her jokes—not "dirty ones," she assured me. She always made "the girls," the aides, laugh. She urged the aides and the housekeeping staff to get an education and make something of their lives.

Just before she had her stroke, she and her husband had to have their beloved dog put down. "I buried her in the fields, so I could look out the window at her," she said.

I told her I would have to be going, I had a plane to catch.

"I've spoken at the state legislature," she responded. She had testified about a land dispute.

She taught vacation Bible school in the summers. Everyone always knew when Jean was teaching, because of the art the children created. "You'd be surprised what you can do with a toothbrush," she said. "You can make spatters like snow."

"I really must go," I said.

"When I worked at Shaw's, I worked the evening shift. When I came home, our youngest would want to go out in the snow. My husband and I bundled her up and put her between us on the snowboard." The moonlight shone on the snowy hills. Below them, the lights from the power plant glowed. It was beautiful.

"I wish I wasn't like this," she said very softly, finally returning to the present day. "I've had a hard time to accept it."

I told her I wished I could stay for hours and hear her stories, but that I had to drive to Manchester or I would miss my plane. I backed out of the room, waving to her, as she continued to talk. "I picked strawberries. For money. For my children's teeth."

Then she waved back at me and said, "Have a good flight."

I so admired Jean for refusing to be defined by her physical condition or by her status of "nursing home resident." She epitomized what researcher Sharon R. Kaufman describes as "the ageless self." In her book of that title, Kaufman explains that people do not find meaning in growing old per se. "To the contrary, when old people talk about themselves, they express a sense of self that is ageless—an identity that maintains continuity despite the physical and social changes that come with old age." She continues, "Old people do not perceive meaning in aging itself, so much as they perceive meaning in being themselves in old age."[1]

I often encountered this deep desire by residents to be known for who they are underneath their disability or age. Family members, too, want people to see their loved ones as individuals whose lives have meant something. Barbara was a round-faced woman with short curly hair and a sweet smile who had experienced a sudden onset of dementia. Her husband immediately let me know that his wife had done important things with her life. As soon as I entered the room, he reached for a news clipping from twenty years earlier. "She founded Helping Hands," he said proudly. "She got her degree in human services."

The chance to hear the life stories of older people is one reason Dr. Martha Stitelman went into geriatrics. She regrets that so much of her time goes to tending to her patients' medical needs that she is often unable to listen to their stories. "It's sad when I read an obituary of someone I took care of for years and I realize what I'd missed," she said. She particularly enjoyed working at the Veterans Administration home, where she found many characters with a sense of humor. Because of the excellent federal benefits, the staff had little turnover and had forged strong bonds with the veterans. "They really got to know the guys who lived there very well," she said. "The vets, tough old birds, were not about to let anybody shove them around, either. They had a smoking lounge, they drank as much beer as they wanted, and they had a pool table that workers played with them."

Having the chance to hear and to tell life stories has long been recognized as a path toward personal growth. In the 1960s, for example, renowned gerontologist Robert Butler, MD, used the life-review process in his therapy work to help people deal with unresolved guilt and grief.

In his extensive research on creativity and aging, Gene Cohen, MD, of George Washington University found that life stories are powerful both for the individuals who tell them and for those who hear them. "The external process of sharing our experiences and telling what we know enables us to combine qualities of creativity and aging to become *keepers of the culture,* the long recognized role of elders, passing on values, wisdom, and a way of life, whether in the culture of a family, a geographic community, or a people bound by ideology," he wrote in *The Creative Age* (emphasis his).[2] Beyond this, Dr. Cohen notes, telling our life stories is a way to illuminate our identity or sense of self.

In his later work, *The Mature Mind,* Dr. Cohen found that the desire to tell one's story, to take stock, to discern meaning, was a nearly universal part of the experience of aging. Whether through keeping scrapbooks, writing memoirs, telling stories, or reminiscing, older people in all cultures found pleasure and meaning in sharing their life experience.

Providing older people opportunities to tell their stories is a simple, valuable way to add meaning to the later part of life, no matter the setting. These stories help bond staff to residents, as at Wesley Village (see Chapter 6). Dr. Cohen suggests that family members, staff, or volunteers help residents create video biographies as a way to engage multiple generations. Photos and favorite music trigger memories, even in people with dementia. "These provide wonderful opportunities for sharing time together," he told me. "It structures the time. You can go and look at pictures together that have been meaningful and include commentary that others provide. Even a visitor, a volunteer who has never met the individual, can sit and watch these videos with the resident and hear all this information, freeze-frame it, tap into a pocket of memory, and focus more on it. You can be very creative."

In Wisconsin, nursing home residents and community-living elders shared their memories of World War II with nursing students. "When people hear about the project, they ask what it has to do with nursing," said Lois Taft, associate professor of nursing systems and the research team's leader. "It changes the way we practice nursing because the experience changes us as caregivers. The project challenges young nursing students to adjust their attitudes toward older people and appreciate them for the lives they've led rather than focusing on their disabilities. It builds relationships between older adults and caregivers."[3]

Making Art

In her work with clients, my friend Karen Gallant, a creativity coach in Maryland, uses life stories and artistic expression to help people experience themselves as creative beings. Karen works with a wide range of people, including those who are homeless, cancer patients, adolescents, and older people in assisted living and adult day care, to develop their capacity for creativity, which she believes is universal. "I don't believe our creativity capacity diminishes," she said. "It is a little bit harder to access as we grow older. As soon as you access even a tiny spark of it, though, it glows with the brilliance of the whole person. It's still absolutely intact."

Karen uses creative expression to help people transitioning from their own homes to assisted living. In one project, she asked people to visualize a favorite childhood memory and then create a collage, using magazine pictures, feathers, fabric, and other materials. Participants created a name for the collage and told others the story that prompted it. One woman, "Juanita," had significant dementia, but she beamed as she shared her creation of bright flowers and feathers. She spoke of her mother's flower garden and of a hummingbird that came there. As she told the story, she mimicked the hummingbird's call. "Everybody laughed, and she told the whole story again. It was just wonderful. The other people in the group responded and talked about what a beautiful story it was," Karen said.

A pilot project looking at how art might help people with early to mid Alzheimer's disease had equally positive results. Among the findings: 83 percent of the forty-one participants sustained attention for thirty to forty-five minutes; 80 percent expressed pleasure through their relaxed body language, smiles, and laughter; and 78 percent "nonverbally expressed pride." Participants made comments such as, "This gives my hand such pleasure" and "In here I feel like a person again."[4]

A nursing home in Pennsylvania began a continuing, rotating art museum for local artists. Residents organized and curated the shows, developed publicity materials, and helped hang the art. They also helped bake cookies to raise money for special lighting for the gallery. "They were engaging seniors in productive, valuable, meaningful activities," said Nancy Zweibel, senior program officer for the Retirement Research Foundation. "Nursing homes need to open the doors and not do patronizing activities."

At the Mount, artist Bridget Daly runs an art studio and holds weekly classes both for residents and for residents and children together. She encourages people to invest themselves in their artwork. "Their idea of art is da Vinci or Norman Rockwell," she said. "I expose them to different kinds of art—older artists, people of color. I show how Georgia O'Keeffe did more abstract art as she grew older. We have a show every year, where we show one piece from each person. They almost all sell. This validates their worth and gives them positive reinforcement. The message is more important than the media."

At the class I attended, a half-dozen elders came, most of them in wheelchairs. None of them had done art before Bridget had introduced them to it. One woman painted everything she could, including a napkin. Bridget asked her the title of her picture. She pondered it and said, "Birds of a Feather." Two other women, both named Dorothy, said they loved the opportunity to explore art. "I just never thought I could do it," said one. She said her daughter is surprised at what she creates. "I told her, maybe I'll be like that lady who started painting when she was eighty." Grandma Moses? I asked. Yes, she said, smiling.

One man had grown so enthusiastic about his art that his wife had purchased a satchel of supplies that he carried with him. Another regular was not there that day because he had to be with his daughter. Bridget said he was disappointed to miss even one class. He asked Bridget, "Why did my daughter have her surgery scheduled on art day?"

Activities

In the 1960s, Herbert Shore wrote: "The success of any 'program' must be placed in the context of what is meaningful, appropriate, and dignified to the older person."

Gay Hanna, who heads the Society for Arts in Healthcare, had a discouraging experience when her late mother was in the best nursing home money could buy, according to Gay. "If that was the best, I fear for what is the worst," she said. Much of Gay's frustration came from the lack of meaningful activity for people who lived there. "I find these places that have a budget hire the canned musicians. Or recreational therapists have such low expectations," she said. "My mother refused to bounce the balloon."

Only by rescuing her once a month and taking her out on long drives through Virginia did Gay discover that her mother had a new love—opera. From then on, Gay brought her mother opera CDs, a real source of pleasure in her last year of life.

Susan Johnson, a geriatric-care manager in Bethesda, Maryland, also believes that residents' capabilities are sometimes underestimated. At a home for people with Alzheimer's disease that had an excellent reputation, she noticed that listed on the weekly calendar was "bread baking."

"I thought, that's a good activity—kneading the bread, tasting it, smelling it," she said. She happened to be there at the appointed time, but there was no bread baking. She asked if it had been canceled. "In fact, everyone was sitting around not doing anything," she said. "The activities director said, 'Our clients taste and smell it. They don't do the activity. These people are too far gone to be able to participate in making the bread.'"

"That's not an activity," Johnson said to me. "That's a morning snack. That appalled me. It's pretty pathetic. That was from the head of activities. What two-year-old do you know couldn't help bake bread?"

Invariably, a home's activities schedule includes bingo, sing-a-longs, holiday crafts, and entertainment by guest musicians or children's groups. (Bingo, for the uninitiated, seems to be an addictive activity for many residents, who played it long before they moved to the nursing home. When I asked a group of women at Pleasant View what they would change about life there, the first thing they said was, "Bingo is too short.") Sometimes activities are infantilized. A nurse at one home complained to me that at Halloween, aides gave residents small bags of candy, as if they were trick-or-treaters. Why not have children come instead, she wondered, and let the residents pass out the candy themselves, a normal adult role?

Often the scheduled activities do not engage residents, despite the best efforts of staff. A study in the *Journal of Advanced Nursing* found it "interesting" that, "given the time and energy devoted to organized social activities in the nursing home, social activities were mentioned only twice" by residents who were asked what they found helpful in the way of social support.[5]

In *It Shouldn't Be This Way*, a chronicle of their mother's journey through the long-term care system, Robert L. Kane and Joan C. West describe the frustration they felt at these prescribed events.

> On Ruth's bulletin board a weekly calendar of activities was posted, and early in her stay we noted that a current events discussion was being held and suggested that she might like to attend. Joan wheeled her down to what looked like a small gymnasium where an activities person was lining up her audience. Because each attendee had to be brought down by either family or a staff member, it took over half an hour just to gather the participants. The first step in the already delayed process was to take attendance. If Ruth was mildly interested at the initial idea, she lost interest by the time the activity got under way. . . .
>
> None of the participants had chosen the activity and if taking attendance were really necessary, it could have been done more efficiently. Indeed, large group activities attended by heterogeneous collections of residents are poor substitutes for meaningful activity. Real activities need to be tailored to the interests and tolerance of the audience, and they need to engage the residents more actively.[6]

Activities are not about filling up the hours between meals and before bedtime. They represent whether the day—and by extension the lives of residents—has meaning. "An existential vacuum results when a lack of meaning or purpose in one's life is experienced," observes nursing researcher Patricia Burbank. In her article on assessing the meaning of life in older clients, she notes the correlation between purpose in life and physical health status. Not surprisingly, those who feel their lives have no meaning are at risk of depression, among other ailments.[7] Most of the elders in her study ranked relationships as the most important source of meaning in their lives. But Burbank stresses that what constitutes meaning and purpose differs from individual to individual. In the case of a nursing home, only by gleaning from each resident (or family surrogate) what is meaningful can relevant activities be planned.

"By stepping over the threshold into Providence Mount Saint Vincent, people's lives are still important," said Bernice Grieve, a former employee turned resident of the Mount. "To be given a purpose for being here today is important, to live in dignity, to have meaning."

Cathy Butler, sixty-one, was young for a nursing home resident. She and her mother both live at the Mount. Cathy had been disabled all her life and in recent years had suffered numerous medical complications.

The afternoon I was there, midway through watching a video on culture change with administrator Charlene Boyd and me, Cathy excused herself. Her day was full, and she couldn't carve out time to watch the whole program. She needed to go to the art studio to work on framing her photographs, which would be in a show there the following month. Then she had some work on her computer to do, followed by dinner with a friend.

After checking for Cathy in her room a few times, I finally caught up with her that evening. A large, long-haired tiger cat stalked out of the room and glared at me. He had adopted her, she said, and chosen her bed as his own.

"I've been in three nursing homes, ranging from hellish to average," she told me. "Then . . . here." With these last words, she spread her arms to encompass her surroundings at the Mount and a look of joy came over her face. "Two years ago, I woke up every morning asking myself, 'What will become of me?'" she said. "Today I wake up trying to decide which of the people I love here will I get to see today."

As Cathy demonstrated, the best activities are those that a given individual finds truly satisfying.

At Teresian House, an activity might be singing at mass on Sundays. Residents don robes and join in familiar hymns. They do not have to come to rehearsals, and they may even fall asleep during the service, but the point is that they have the chance to participate in a valued ritual and make a contribution, as best they can.

At a Pioneer Network conference, workshop leader Virginia Bell, herself an elder and the coauthor of *The Best Friends Staff: Building a Culture of Care in Alzheimer's Programs*, urged participants to think of activities in a much more organic, natural way than characterizes those typically listed on a schedule. "Older people and people with dementia need someone to make them feel connected, feel loved, feel respected," she said. "Whenever we do that, we do an activity." Her list of twenty simple activities, which she offered to the group from the point of view of a nursing home resident, included such things as "laugh with me—it says someone thinks everything is okay; give me hugs—hugging is a wonderful activity much better than most activities we have; let me show you; let me teach you; ask me for an opinion; invite me to help you," and so on. "One thing that has been such a surprise is people who don't know what day it is still know a lot," she said of her work with people with dementia. For example, one woman with dementia was able to teach a group sign language.

Giving Back

In his book *Dementia Reconsidered*, Tom Kitwood discusses ten positive types of interaction that support a high quality of life for people with cognitive impairment. Nursing homes typically overlook one of these, collaboration. "The hallmark of collaboration is that care is not something that is 'done to' a person who is cast into a passive role; it is a process in which their own initiative and abilities are involved," Kitwood noted.[8] In a nursing home, and in society in general, frail elders are most often on the receiving end of a relationship. But the duality of being cared for and caring for others is intrinsic to our sense of well-being.

As culture-change expert and psychologist Judah Ronch writes: "Humanization can occur only when caregiver-recipient relationships define the quality of care. Simply stated, an I-thou relationship is a significant source of clinical benefit for the resident and a significant source of job satisfaction for the employee because it considers the needs, concerns, and characteristics of the care recipient as well as the caregiver to be the foundation of a mutually enriching relationship."[9] No matter the age, giving help—rather than receiving it—is associated with higher levels of mental well-being.

I thought of Louisa, an upbeat woman at Pleasant View who gets around in an electric wheelchair without which she would go crazy, she told me. She is Greek American, and her family owned a successful diner in Concord, where she also worked when she was younger. When I asked about her life at the nursing home, the first thing she mentioned was not her aches and pains, the food, or waiting for call lights to be answered—it was a service project she helped organize as copresident of Pleasant View's community council. The group raffles holiday baskets at Valentine's Day and Thanksgiving and raises money to donate to a charity. The baskets, filled with such things as coupons for gasoline, an oven mitt, candy, and stationery, can raise as much as three to four hundred dollars. Louisa spoke of a resident who had since died who made beautiful greeting cards that the group sold. Louisa also had a telephone—not a given in a nursing home—which she used not only to talk to her large family but also to perform volunteer work for her church, helping to organize contributions for a local food pantry.

Like her sister Pleasant View resident, Jean, Louisa refused to be defined by the setting in which she found herself. She had given to others all her life, and she had found a way to continue to serve. She was hardly a Pollyanna, but she lived with grace and dignity. "I don't think you ever get adjusted [to living in a nursing home]," she said, "but you do the best you can. The worst part is waiting for someone to help you. Or for a man to bathe you or put you to bed. I refuse to let a man do that."

At Ridgewood Center in Bedford, New Hampshire, community service projects linked everyone. For a local food drive, not only did staff and family contribute, but residents were taken shopping so that they could buy food to contribute.

Women in the Green House in Tupelo, who had been homemakers all their lives continued as best they could, setting the table, doing laundry, sharing recipes, helping cook, hugging a child. At the Mount, in Seattle, a group of very old women, some with shaking hands and very poor eyesight, sat around a dining table, hulling strawberries. There was a pleasant ordinariness to the task. I could imagine these women working on a covered-dish supper at church or sitting on the front porch together on a summer day.

At Thanksgiving, the staff of one neighborhood at the Mount decided it would be fun to cook a real homemade dinner. "I wanted them to smell pies baking and turkey roasting," said Brenda Jennings, the neighborhood coordinator. "One of my ladies snapped beans forever."

The staff polled the residents to learn their favorite dishes. One remembered having plum pudding at Christmastime. As a child, she came home from school and stirred the pudding and made a wish. Brenda joked that they almost burned the place down trying to make the pudding flambé, as the resident remembered. "But the look on her face was worth it," she said.

Simply helping each other is meaningful. In a study of social support, residents spoke of the support they gave other residents, such as rubbing the hands of someone whose hands were cold, sharing a pack of cigarettes, walking and talking together, assisting someone at mealtime.[10] Such mutual support can also link people across the spectrum of a continuing-care retirement community.

At Lenawee nursing home in Adrian, Michigan, I met Mr. Lewis, who had recently been moved to a newly renovated wing. To me, the wing seemed much nicer than the others, especially because of the private rooms. Mr. Lewis had a white dove in a cage and had filled his room with a profusion of plants that he propagated. He had on a work shirt and jeans and used an oxygen machine. As I admired his room, he told me that he missed his old room. I asked why, and he said he missed looking after his roommate. "Helping someone else does more good than any medicine," he told me.

Those who have dementia also welcome opportunities to give. In his discussion of a writing group for people with dementia, psychologist Alan Dienstag notes that not only did their writing preserve memories, but listening to each other's stories was reward in itself for participants. "Alzheimer's disease is an illness in which the losses accumulate moment by moment and day by day," he wrote. "Giving reverses the tide and represents a refusal to be defined by loss."[11]

Besides giving to others, people in nursing homes find meaning in exerting their independence and self-reliance. By taking care of their own needs as best they can, residents retain dignity and have the satisfaction of not burdening overworked aides. Ruth, at Pleasant View, took obvious pride in doing for herself as much as she could. She was responsible for taking her medications, and every morning an aide brought her a basin of hot water so she could take care of her own washing routine. Ruth also took pride in being able to laugh at life's challenges. She regaled me with stories of roommates come and gone. Where others might be angry or irritated, Ruth found humor. "I remember one roommate who they told me was very sweet and soft-spoken. The first night she stayed in here, I was sound asleep and I hear someone yell, "Nurse!" Here, Ruth let out a bellow. "She sounded like a foghorn!"

Ruth did not minimize the difficulties of life at Pleasant View. But she was both stoic and philosophical. "There is a great deal of turnover," she said. "You see things you don't want to see. But they happen, and you have to face life."

I asked her what she thinks the public needs to understand about life in a nursing home. "Nursing homes are not where you come to die," she said. "It's where you come to live. You're not alone, all in a muddle. There's someone caring for you. If you fall, someone will help you. Look at how many people come in! Their lives can change and broaden, and they come alive again. If you think of the old concept, where you're sick and you go there to die—that's not the way it is today, and it shouldn't be that way."

Nurturing Life

There is something inherently hopeful about gardening. Not only is the work of planting satisfying, so is the faith that the seeds will grow and bring fruit or flower. When our friend Annie Lustig, forty-one, had brain cancer, she asked her friends to help plant bulbs in her family's yard in the autumn. We all pitched in. She never got to see them bloom, but her fierce hopefulness moved all of us.

"When spring comes I'll be so glad," Louisa, at Pleasant View, told me. "We have a garden in the back, and we help collect tomatoes, cucumbers, and squash."

As Bill Thomas explains in *Life Worth Living*, his book on the Eden Alternative, the opportunity to nurture life is deeply satisfying, no matter our age or condition. Although only a handful of nursing home residents may be physically able to actively garden, many can participate in smaller tasks—starting seeds, transplanting seedlings, or making use of the garden's products. "At the very least, they will enjoy the colors and scents and take pleasure in eating fresh, truly homegrown food," he writes.

At Oatfield Estates, outside Portland, Oregon, organic gardening is an integral part of life. Oatfield Estates sits atop a hill, and from the grounds, you can enjoy breathtaking views of snow-peaked Mount Hood and Mount Jackson. In January, the garden beds had only brown stalks but I was told repeatedly of the bounty of flowers and vegetables they would yield. Residents, many with dementia, had just finished poring over seed catalogues, making their selection for the spring planting. Large, raised beds allow them to work in the garden, even if they are in wheelchairs. Each household's chef uses the fresh produce that residents harvest. More than two-thirds of the residents participate in gardening.

Oatfield Estates encourages people to help out in all sorts of ways. One man enjoyed being the maintenance man's assistant. Another regularly loaded the dishwasher. A woman peeled carrots.

Many of the homes I visited allowed residents to bring pets with them when they moved in and encouraged staff to bring their dogs to work each day. Other homes had adopted cats, dogs, or birds that became part of the life of the community. Seeing a cat stalk silently down the halls of a nursing home, or a little dog hopeful for a pat on the head, always made me smile.

There are many examples, both in pet therapy literature and my own visits, of animals as a bridge between isolated, noncommunicative residents and the rest of the community. As we have seen, a woman at Spruce Lodge in Bigfork began eating again and engaging with others after she was befriended by the white cat, Wilfred. In *Between Pets and People*, Alan Beck and Aaron Katcher describe Jed, who had lived in a nursing home in Ohio for twenty-six years after suffering brain damage in a fall. No one thought he could hear or speak. After a pet-therapy program was introduced, Jed was transformed. The first time Jed saw the dog Whiskey, he spoke: "You brought that dog." From then on, he began talking again, his mood improved, and he produced copious drawings of dogs.[12] A small body of research looks at the people-pet connection. Although the mechanisms are not understood, caring for pets is associated with reducing stress, lowering blood pressure, and reducing depression, among other benefits.

Fostering Hope

Older people, at least as much as the general population, are religious. Nine out of ten believe in God and pray regularly. A study by Harold Koenig, MD, and his colleagues found that nearly 60 percent of nursing home residents used religion to help them cope. This study confirms many others that show people dealing with chronic illness are able to cope better if they are religious. Religious belief may buffer people against the ill effects of stress that comes from debilitating illness.[13] For example, a study of elderly women recovering from hip fractures found that those with strong religious beliefs and practices were less depressed and could walk farther at the time of discharge.[14]

Reviews of the literature show a consistent association between religiosity and better mental health and social support. Nursing researcher Theris A. Touhy cited a qualitative study of a nursing home that found "the presence of affirming spiritual beliefs and practices was identified by all but one of the 60 participants as important in fostering hope."[15]

A study of sixty-nine older residents from nine nursing homes in Florida found no significant differences in their level of hope based on factors such as physical health, education, functional ability, or age. But there was a significant correlation between spirituality and level of hope. Touhy strongly urged nurses to intentionally address spiritual concerns of nursing home residents. "Limiting care to only physical needs denies elders the opportunity to live out their lives with meaning, purpose and hope," wrote Touhy.[16]

Similarly, a number of common themes emerged in a study in which ninety-five residents of six long-term care facilities were asked open-ended questions about what behaviors kept them as healthy as possible. "Feeling valued by self and others is important; responding to the needs of others can facilitate transcending tremendous losses; love and the memory of love continue to have meaning; keeping mind, body, and spirit active gives meaning to life; and a belief in God or higher power gives meaning to suffering and loss."[17]

Yet nursing homes rarely address the religious or spiritual needs of either residents or staff, who must regularly deal with death and dying. "Nursing homes typically don't have chaplains, and pastors and priests typically don't visit people in nursing homes, so there is no one to help them with their spiritual needs," according to Dr. Koenig.[18] He suggests an affordable way to address nursing home residents' spiritual needs: Train volunteer laypeople in clinical pastoral education.

Faith-based homes I visited seemed particularly comfortable with addressing residents' spiritual needs. As Rev. Garth Brokaw of Fairport Baptist put it, "I've always said that it's probably more important for someone to go to chapel than it is to have a bath."

At Wesley Village, Rev. Jim Stinson, director of spiritual life, pays attention to the spiritual needs of residents and staff alike. Noting that the Planetree model includes spirituality as one of ten key components, he said, "I have always believed if we aren't creating environments for healthy relationships, nobody is going to be spiritually whole, and they won't feel good."

Every year, the Wesley Village community has a spring renewal event for staff, residents, and families. There has been a drumming circle where everyone plays music together, a maypole celebration, a jazz quartet, and a "village soup" that residents help make. "We tell the Planetree story," said Rev. Stinson. "It's all held outdoors and there's music. For me, that's part of the spiritual piece. Our goal is to have people understand [the nursing home] might be their last physical stop, but it's not the end of their life."

Another ritual is a "blessing of the hands" for staff. Half the staff participate in the voluntary activity. Using aromatic oils, Rev. Stinson talks to the staff about how their hands are needed in the ministry of healing. He starts with one person and says, "May your hands be hands of blessing in the years to come." The blessing is repeated, from one person to the next, until everyone has received it. When some of the residents heard of the blessing, they asked to participate as well. "It's a way of reminding them they still have something to contribute to this world," he said.

The Mount is also extraordinary in addressing spiritual needs. Because the building was formerly a convent, its chapel is impressive, with frosted-glass windows and statuary. Mass is held nearly every morning, and some of the residents who seem the worst off regularly attend. I slipped in for a few moments of peace and serenity. A sister made many trips down the hall, wheeling in residents for mass. "Do you want some holy water, Katy?" she asked a woman. When she assented, the nun gently guided the woman's hand to the basin of water.

Nursing Home

by Lillian Morrison

My mother is all bones
and eyes.
She doesn't notice
her clothes anymore
who had loved beads and bright colors
or glance at the racketing dayroom TV
who had watched her "stories" every day.
"These are my company."
Just people she wants
to greet and joke with,
to cry a little.
She wants them to smile
and to love her.
She asks for her father and mother.
I touch the baby skin,
the meaningful face
and look in the eyes that say
"I'm still fighting
in this narrow place."
and I hug
the fragile bones.

  —Reprinted with permission of the author

In every nursing home are many people who seem "too far gone" to partake in life in a way that the rest of us would find meaningful. In my conversation with Dr. Martha Stitelman, she asked, "What is the role of the oldest old? When is the time to make a legacy, and when is the time to say good-bye? Some are not still growing and some are not creating meaning for themselves."

These are difficult questions, with no simple answers. But in all these examples—hugging and being hugged, stroking a cat, smiling at a child, smelling home cooking, listening to a favorite piece of music—there is meaning and pleasure, no matter how ill and frail we have become.

"We think people who can't communicate or who are debilitated don't have anything going on inside of them," said Christa Hojlo of the Veterans Administration. "I firmly believe we all do, until we're dead. Why should we be satisfied with allowing a human being to vegetate? My staff will say, 'They don't want to get out of bed. They want to stay in their pajamas. That's a resident's right.' It's not. They don't have a right to vegetate. If we think it's okay for them to choose to lie in bed day after day, that is our problem—we have given them no reason to get out of bed."

Those in the Pioneer Network maintain that until the point of death, we are growing, vital individuals. As nursing home maverick Carter Williams has written:

The days of our lives, even the days and years in a nursing home, are for living, not merely for physical safekeeping. They are days for nurture of mind and spirit as well as body, and for the richness of community. To *live* these days in all their potential it is necessary for all of us to be known and responded to as individual people who have life experiences and daily patterns of many sorts, who are constitutionally different one from another, and who therefore have different sources of meaning in our later years. In order to be people that matter, to be of account to others as we have known ourselves to be at other ages and states of wellness, we must be heard and responded to individually as we try to make sense of our daily lives.[19]

Chapter 9

Family-Friendly Homes
Welcoming Relatives to the Team

Be nice to your children—they'll be choosing
your nursing home
            —Bumper sticker in Maryland, 2004

Americans are just too busy, and here's proof: They can pay
a new business to visit relatives in the nursing home. . . . We
don't know what the fees are, but there's something cold and
distant about saying, in effect, "Here's 20 bucks. Go visit my
grandma."
            —Editorial, the *Toledo (Ohio) Blade,* May 9, 2006

We must move away from the position which views family
interest and concern as interference, away from a position
that is suspicious and resentful of family, to one which
creates a true spirit of sharing and cooperation.
            —Herbert Shore, "New Ideas in Institutional Care"

Ellen Proxmire, whose husband, the late senator William Proxmire, had
Alzheimer's disease, described how it felt to be thrust into the role
of caregiver. "The hardest thing is you can't believe this is happening," she
said. "It affects your friendships. People don't want to deal with it. Money
becomes an issue. It's terribly expensive, and it's too late to get long-term
care insurance. You're facing dealing with this on a daily basis. It's hard to
sleep. It's hard to plan."

Her anguish was not unusual. Families are left to their own devices to
handle incredibly complex burdens. Your time is no longer your own, as you
sublimate your own wants and needs. Simple pleasures you have long taken

for granted—eating at a restaurant, going to a movie, planning a vacation—go by the wayside. You may have to administer complicated medication regimes, give injections or other unpleasant treatments, or help bathe, dress, and feed your loved one. Family roles often reverse. Children must look out for parents. Spouses take over household responsibilities—cooking, cleaning, car repair, home maintenance—that have long been performed by their husband or wife. Life becomes an endless series of medical appointments. You feel lonely. Old friends call less and less. They don't know what to say. The help you need, to give you a break, you often cannot afford. You live in a constant state of stress, and your own health may deteriorate.

"The problem is not that public policy looks first to families but that it generally looks only to families and fails to support those who accept responsibility," writes Carol Levine in "The Loneliness of the Long-Term Care Giver."[1]

Levine herself is a caregiver for her husband who, at sixty-two was in a serious automobile accident that left him with major brain damage. In addition to her full-time job with the United Hospital Fund in New York, she is his care manager, a task that requires "grit and persistence," she writes, not to mention considerable money to pay for daytime aides, prescription drugs, medical devices and supplies, and many other expenses.

Thus it is all the more impressive to realize that not professionals but family members provide most caregiving of elders in our society, and indeed around the world. In the United States, some 44 to 50 million people are caregivers, representing 21 percent of all households. Families contribute an estimated $257 billion worth of unpaid care to loved ones each year.[2]

The recipients of this care, typically older widows, may need help with weekly errands or bill paying, or they may require full-time assistance with bathing, dressing, and eating. In their survey of family caregiving, the National Alliance for Caregiving and AARP found that 25 percent of people who need care live with their caregivers, usually their children, while 55 percent still live in their own homes, 5 percent live in a nursing home, and 4 percent live in assisted living.

Family members who care for relatives with Alzheimer's disease carry the heaviest burden, both physically and emotionally. Two-thirds of these caregivers have had to miss work because of their caregiving responsibilities. Nearly half gave up vacations, hobbies, or social activities, and 40 percent reported high levels of emotional stress.[3]

Caregiving can also divide families, as siblings rarely share duties equally. Some may think Mom would be better off with paid caregivers in a facility, for example, while others are reluctant to see that care eat up their inheritance.

Even though caregiving can be painful, difficult, and terribly lonely, family members express a deep sense of satisfaction about their role and feel proud of giving loving care. "Some see it as a means to give back to loved ones who have cared for them so well in the past," notes psychologist Barry Jacobs.[4]

Making the Move

Many families, though, try as they might, are unable to provide all the services and care their loved ones need. They make the difficult decision to move them to long-term care. Usually this move is a wrenching one. "I just hated the thought—I still do," said Ellen Proxmire. "But Bill was in danger constantly. He would disappear." She had the wherewithal to visit twenty facilities before finding one that she felt provided good care. "I'm comforted that he's here, and I feel fortunate—it's very expensive," she said in an interview with me before his death.

Even in this situation, Ellen Proxmire, like most family members, said she regretted that she was unable to care for her husband at home. "You resist it to the end," she said. "You feel guilty, sad, beleaguered, angry, inadequate. It's a sea of conflict and it never goes away."

Often a medical crisis forces the decision, allowing little time for preparation or for researching the best facilities. Family members may feel they've failed, or they question their priorities. Are they putting their work or other loved ones' needs above their parents'?

Rarely do families "dump" their relatives in nursing homes to relieve themselves of the caregiving burden. In fact, many caregivers continue to experience stress and disruption after their relatives move. Time pressures shift to a heavy visiting schedule, with family visits or phone calls averaging more than four hours a week.[5]

Family caregivers spend money, as well as time and energy. On average, they spend approximately five hundred dollars a month out of pocket toward resident care in nursing homes (four hundred a month for those in assisted living) for transportation and extra services not included in the facility fees.[6]

Although many families visit regularly for years on end, others do not. One study found that visits dropped off soon after the family member made the move. "Perhaps the most striking finding . . . is that, although families tend to live quite close to their loved one in a nursing home, contact via in-person visits and telephone calls dropped by approximately half within the first few weeks and months of placement."[7] This study identified logistical problems that hinder low-income families from visiting. The authors suggested organizing volunteer transportation pools, offering family caregivers flextime at work, and addressing health and psychological needs of family members as ways to encourage more visiting.

There may be another reason family visits flag. Visiting in a nursing home can be excruciating. Family members and friends do not know what to do with themselves. One study found that many families "sat and stared at their relative for an hour twice a week," unsure of how to relate to them. "As a result, very few family members actually looked forward to visiting. Instead, visiting was associated with feelings of frustration, anger, resentment, and guilt."[8]

As noted earlier, many nursing homes do not have pleasant, private places for families to spend time together. In a barren environment, there is little to distract or engage you. With many residents suffering depression or cognitive impairment, normal conversation can be halting. Children will be bored or frightened and may dread visiting Grandma.

Moreover, family members often feel unwelcome, not only because of the physical environment, but because of the attitude of employees. A chasm of mistrust and miscommunication often divides families and nursing home staff. Families struggling to advocate for their loved ones nearly always are unhappy about something, from missing laundry, hearing aids, or dentures, to slow response to call lights. Even at the most expensive homes, families complain of poor care, callous staff, and defensive administrators. Racial, ethnic, or language differences between families and aides can further complicate already difficult relationships.

Almost every time I write about long-term care, I receive e-mails from family members who want to share upsetting experiences, such as this one:

> Since my mom had her stroke in August life has been a nightmare. We have found that the word 'care' no longer means thoughtful, kind, with a smile. It is reduced to folks just showing up to get a paycheck. My mom spent 2 months in a place that was never cleaned (unless my sister and I did it—which we did daily); we found poop on the floor; dirty toilet paper on the back of the toilet; on two occasions we found poop on mom's legs; we found her early one morning with her feeding tube connected wrong and all her food was soaked into the bedding, her clothes. All the administration did was blame us. They even went so far as to call a meeting with us. . . . When we got to the meeting, the amount of people we were told were going to be there was doubled (they even brought their attorney) and it was to point fingers at my dad, not to discuss the care.

The National Citizens' Coalition for Nursing Home Reform, as well as geriatric-care managers and state ombudsmen, strongly urge family involvement as the best way to protect nursing home residents from such neglect. Family members, imbued with a lifetime of horror stories about nursing homes, may come armed with suspicion and determined to demand the good care their loved ones deserve.

My friend Sara described an incident at a rehabilitation center where her mother was staying. The center was clean and seemed to be well run. But the staff was unfriendly. Sara did her best to win them over, making requests in a pleasant manner and even baking them cookies. But she always felt a wall of indifference or even hostility. When she requested a care-planning meeting, the staff was defensive, despite the decades-long mandate from the Nursing Home Reform Law that residents and family members be actively involved in care planning. During the meeting, the staff stood with arms crossed, treating Sara as an adversary.

Sara was experiencing what studies have found: Nursing home staff generally do not see family members as part of the caregiving team. Instead, they view families either as complaining, picky, and unappreciative, or as absent and uncaring. Families don't understand what is best for their loved one. They expect miracles. They are dysfunctional.

"When I go out to speak, I ask how many people [who work in nursing homes] are not having any problems with family members—and you can hear the laughter around the hall," said Rose Marie Fagan, director of the Pioneer Network.

This family-staff tension may be a carryover from the hospital model, itself flawed, as described by Planetree in its book on transforming to a patient-centered care model:

> Many staff members and physicians feel that families are dysfunctional when family members question staff actions or persist in trying to meet patient demands. When hospital staff members are asked to list the attributes of the "perfect patient and family," their response is usually a passive patient with no family. The ideal patient is described as one who does not ask questions, never rings the call bell, does exactly what he or she is told, and has no visible family members or friends to advocate on his or her behalf. Which is more "dysfunctional"—the family trying to support their loved one or the staff member who pretends they don't exist and aren't important?[9]

In fact, what families say they want is pretty basic. They want their loved ones to be given kind and courteous care. They wanted staff to address them by name, and they would like their own contributions acknowledged rather than rebuffed. They want to be kept informed about their relative's condition, and they want to feel part of a caregiving team. They want to feel that staff members have personal knowledge of their loved one and actually enjoy being around older people. Of course none of this is possible if aides are constantly being pulled from floor to floor, calling in sick, or quitting in frustration. In fact, there is a very strong correlation between family satisfaction and employee satisfaction.[10]

Having a good relationship with family members who value their work rather than always finding fault is important to aides. A program called Partners in Caregiving taught staff and families in ten nursing homes new, open ways to communicate and gave each insight into how the others felt. The program had positive outcomes for both, including decreased staff turnover and families forming family councils within the nursing homes.[11]

For residents, visits from family and friends ranks at the top of what is important to them. Those fortunate residents who have regular visitors have less confusion, agitation, depression, regression, and verbal and physical hostility. Family members are a link to the past and remind residents of who they truly are. Families can tell staff what activities, interests, jokes, and idiosyncrasies make up an individual. Imagine yourself living in a "home" with strangers. You are sick or frail or forgetful. Trying to assert your identity and allowing people to know you for the person you have always been would be daunting indeed, especially if you have no loved ones around.

Family members also have an important and little acknowledged role to play in helping staff give better clinical care, especially for residents who have dementia. One study found that family members' intimate knowledge of their relative enabled them to identify breathing and swallowing problems that professional staff had overlooked. "Such refined skills of the family members should not be ignored," the study noted.[12]

Not only do residents feel happier and family members less guilty when communication is open and friendly, but staff and administrators, too, can lower their defenses. The warmer their relationships are with families, the less likely administrators are to receive complaints from ombudsmen and to be sued.

When Steve McAlilly first became an administrator in Mississippi, the number and the intensity of family complaints shocked him. "The nursing home industry said it was all guilt on the part of families, and that their standards were too high," he said. But he was convinced that transforming the culture of the institution would cause family complaints to decline. "We were driven to have a place that families would be proud of and not say a prayer when they entered the nursing home, 'God save me from this.'"

Family-Friendly Homes

Transformational homes are places where families feel welcome and happy to visit. Not that there won't still be problems. For example, some family members may disagree with the idea of not using physical restraints (see Chapter 3). In the film *Almost Home*, which documents one Wisconsin nursing home's culture-change journey, a husband showed little sympathy for resident-directed care. When his wife wanted to sleep late, he accused the aides of being too lazy to get her up. But it's safe to say that once culture change is implemented, most families feel far better about their loved ones living with more dignity and affection.

In the homes I visited, family members I encountered were nearly always pleased with the quality of life and care their relatives were receiving. Wesley Village, for example, as part its relationship-centered approach, drew on Planetree's family-friendly policies. Clarence Canfield, whose wife Esther lived there, was active in the family support group. "I'd never have her anywhere else but here," he said. "This is the friendliest bunch of people. It's true."

He and other family members had a comfortable gathering place, a room with plenty of natural light, armchairs and sofas, and a basket with simple activities and a list of "101 Meaningful Visits." This wonderful resource gives family members who feel awkward or at a loss plenty of ideas of fun, imaginative, and rewarding things to do with loved ones. Among the suggestions: Eat lunch with a resident who has no family visitors, reserve the residents' kitchen to bake a favorite family dessert together, give a hand massage (scented lotions provided), have a wine or cheese tasting, and "listen to the sound machine in the chapel with the lights out."

Bonnie Kantor, director of geriatrics and gerontology at Ohio State University, shared a personal story that exemplified what families want. Her mother had suffered from dementia for years and lived in a nursing home in New York, hundreds of miles away. She didn't speak, got around in a wheelchair, and ate only pureed food. One day, two aides were chatting together about going to Wendy's for lunch.

All of a sudden my mother uttered the first sentence she had said since she'd been there in five years—"Can I go too?" Everything stopped. They said, "Where do you want to go, Miriam?" And she said, "Wendy's." They said to her, "What would you have?" And she said, "Chicken nuggets." Somebody ran over to the head nurse and said, "Can we take Miriam to Wendy's?" This is a woman who hasn't been out of the nursing home, can't walk without incredible assistance—and the nurse said yes.

This was a great example of putting the person before the task. They had to know the next shift wasn't going to mind doing a little more for some people, if they didn't get a bath or something, because everybody would be so excited that Miriam did this.

They got her all dolled up and put her in the car and took her to Wendy's and got carryout. They weren't sure what kind of sauce she wanted, so they got all of them. Meanwhile they called me on a speakerphone in her room, so that I could be part of the party. As her daughter and as a professional, I knew she could die—she was eating chicken nuggets and she's been on a pureed diet. Did they know in twenty minutes she'd have no memory of it? Sure. Did that matter? No. It provided them with a connection, so for the next long time they could say, "Miriam, remember when we went to Wendy's?"

It's not only giving staff the opportunity to develop close relationships that makes homes family friendly. By changing the physical layout and creating more of a home environment, nursing homes also become more welcoming places. In contrast, an institutional hospital design reinforces a sense of awkwardness and not belonging.

For Frances Anglin, having her husband who had severe dementia in a Green House meant a lot, even if he might not fully grasp his surroundings. "It's the families that know the difference," she said. "He can't converse." She appreciated the privacy residents had there. "It's roomier—it seems more like a home than a nursing home. People here are like family. When he sees me, he brightens up." So too did he brighten up when he saw children, she said. Children of staff come frequently to the Green Houses. As we spoke, Vera Laney, an elder for whom the household was named, approached Mrs. Anglin and gave her two big kisses on the cheek.

Transformative homes encourage family members to eat there by not charging them for meals or by providing space for family-style dining. "We encourage families to be part of the communities," said Brenda Jennings at the Mount. "We feed spouses along with everyone else. We have someone whose mom died here, she still comes to help at mealtime."

At Oatfield Estates in Oregon, household chefs had an incentive to invite others to dine: the more people they served, the more their food budget was increased. "They really encourage us to invite extra family and friends," a resident told me. That day a friend was coming to visit her; there were ample areas for the two of them to eat together privately.

Rose Marie Fagan has a wealth of experience, not only as head of the Pioneer Network, but from her earlier career as a long-term care ombudsman and as a family caregiver whose mother had lived at Fairport Baptist Nursing

Home. "That was the beauty here," she said, when we toured Fairport Baptist together, along with administrator Garth Brokaw. "There's an openness and receptiveness to family. There's a natural role that evolves and develops for a family member. The way that plays out is, my mother was living in a household—that's her home. There's a kitchen table, there's coffee going. I stopped in to see her almost every day and she could say, 'Do you want a cup of coffee?' When there was very little to talk to my mother about, I could talk to other residents, family members, staff, because we're all gathered around that kitchen table."

Garth said they saw an "incredible increase" in family participation once they had changed to a household. "They come more, they stay longer, they bring more kids."

"Because there's something to do," Rose Marie said. "You can bring food in, you can have a meal here. You can help with dishes or clear the table if you want to. You can sit and talk to people. You can do your mother's laundry. You just feel a part of it. My husband used to come when my mother had physical therapy. He was able to go with her when she had therapy and cheer her on, which is huge. It's absolutely huge, when I reflect back on that. I've been in nursing homes as an ombudsman where they won't let you anywhere near the physical therapy room."

When I asked her why that would be, she said,

I don't know. I used to challenge it all the time. They'd say it's the rules—"regulations." Here, there was no hassle. We didn't have to ask permission. My husband just showed up, he didn't interfere or anything, he just cheered her on. Or my son used to come. There were people to talk to, and he'd have lunch with her.

I felt like I was still my mother's caregiver. My mother needed some services that I couldn't provide. But I still had my role. Nobody took my role away.

Chapter 10

The Zen of Memory Loss
Living in the Moment

Nora is immobile and, we suppose, demented. She cannot talk or move, though her eyes radiate alertness and joy. Sometimes she smiles and makes musical cooing sounds. Sometimes she laughs softly for no apparent reason. Surely it's her unrelenting contentment and profound happiness that convince us that she must be out of her mind.

> —Tom Gass, *Nobody's Home: Candid Reflections of a Nursing Home Aide*

I've learned an awful lot—like how to take care of people with dementia. I've learned a lot more patience with everybody. I had no idea how to approach somebody with dementia. In fact, I was almost afraid of them. But you treat them with respect and love like anybody else, and they come around to tender loving care.

> —Ida Cummings, Green House shahbaz

My visit to Arbor Place in Rockville, Maryland, was a revelation. As I entered, I heard Latin jazz throbbing. Before me, in the living room, the household was in full swing. A gentleman in a plaid shirt dipped into a romantic embrace with a regal woman wearing a full skirt, her hair tucked into a ballerina's bun. Others held their partners' hands and bobbed to the beat. Some who were in wheelchairs hand-danced with their partners. When the song ended, everyone laughed and hugged. It was hard for me to believe that every resident there had Alzheimer's disease.[1]

"Here, from the time they get up to the time they go to bed, it's about

pleasure," said Eileen Fanburg, who codirects Arbor Place with her husband, geriatric psychiatrist Walter H. Fanburg.

The contrast to most other dementia-care facilities is so striking that family members have been known to burst into tears when they first set foot in the door.

Stephanie Waldron, whose search for alternative living for her mother had left her feeling "desperate," knew instantly that Arbor Place was unusual. "When I first came, I had so much fun here," she told me. "The residents had me in stitches playing a gambling game. When I left here, I felt happy."

The Fanburgs have taken the most advanced thinking on dementia care and applied it to an assisted-living home they created from the ground up. Arbor Place is far more expensive than most families can afford—$261 a day in 2005. But other homes could learn a lot from the quality of life there. According to geriatric-care consultant Susan Johnson, Arbor Place is among the best dementia-care facilities in the country—a "beacon in a sea of mediocrity," as she put it. "If you read the brochures of other places, they all are saying the same thing: good activities, customized care. But they may not deliver on that promise. The Fanburgs deliver. They provide stimulating activities that are for adults, not childlike activities just to keep people busy."

Perhaps even more important, Johnson added, is the opportunity to form meaningful relationships. "That's important for all of us, but especially for people with dementia," she said. "Some of these other places provide shelter and food, but people are not having human interactions and relationships. That's what I'm very impressed with at Arbor Place."

As discussed earlier, roughly half of those in nursing homes and 24 to 42 percent in assisted living have dementia. Some 4.5 million people have Alzheimer's disease in the United States. In 2006, one in three Americans had a family member or friend with Alzheimer's disease. Nationally, the direct and indirect cost of caring for people with Alzheimer's is $100 billion a year.[2]

People with dementia face considerable, progressive losses, as do their families. Bit by bit, memory ebbs away, first in the short term—how to get from your house to the grocery, where you put your purse, when to go to a doctor's appointment—and gradually more and more. Often the person is adept at concealing her confusion for years. If family members begin to question irrational behavior, the person may grow angry or frightened. Eventually, sufferers will not recognize their own spouse or children. They may begin to wander at all hours of the day or night, trying to get to a job they held forty years ago or searching for long-dead parents.

Families find it harder and harder to manage. Yet they often delay moving their loved ones, not only out of guilt and emotional loss, but because finding

a high-quality, affordable home is difficult. When people with Alzheimer's are moved to traditional nursing homes, the institutional atmosphere may aggravate their troubling behavior. The loud beepers and buzzers, disembodied voices over loudspeakers, harried staff, and constantly changing faces are especially jarring for those already confused and frightened.

"We've marginalized people with Alzheimer's and, as a society, relegated them to these archaic ways of providing care," said Sharon Brangman, MD, division chief of geriatrics at SUNY Upstate Medical University in Syracuse and a board member of the American Geriatric Society. "Most people don't want to be in an institutional setting, and most family members don't want to put a loved one in there. There's an increasing interest in looking at care that is organized in a more homelike setting, where activities and medical care are really patient centered rather than on an institutional schedule. The problem is, we still in this country have a mindset that is a very medical model about taking care of people, and it takes a while to get that mindset or culture to change."

A retirement community I visited in the Midwest had built a nice, homey building for people with Alzheimer's. But as their condition worsened, they had to move to the nursing home—a grim fate. I encountered a woman there who epitomized the behavior so dreaded in people with dementia. As I walked by and greeted her, she fiercely grabbed my wrist and would not let go. She told me all manner of horrible things—the staff had kidnapped her granddaughter and had her tied up naked, and so on. I tried my best to reassure her, but I could tell from the look in her eyes that she saw me as part of the evil conspiracy. I managed to extricate myself when someone distracted her, but it was a brief window for me into how scary it would be either to live in this woman's world or to be responsible for her care.

I wondered, though, how much of her anger could be traced to her environment. In such a momentary encounter, I could not say. But even before I met the troubled woman, I wanted to flee. Everything about the place felt wrong. You exited the elevator to face an imposing nurse's station. In the hallways, people sat in wheelchairs with nothing going on to engage them. The atmosphere was stifling, and particularly distressing as I knew this was a place with a good reputation. I felt I would go mad if I had to live there. Why should we expect anything different from residents, whatever their cognitive state?

In recent years, we have learned much about how people with dementia might lead better lives. As British psychologist Tom Kitwood writes in *Dementia Reconsidered*: "Dementia, as a concept, is losing its terrifying associations with the raving lunatic in the old-time asylum. It is being perceived as an understandable and human condition, and those who are affected by it have begun to be recognized, welcomed, embraced and heard."[3] He argues that far too much attention has been devoted to pharmacological fixes, too little to supporting a high quality of life and care.

"The case for better care has become overwhelmingly strong," Kitwood writes. "An ethic of respect for persons requires it. Empirical evidence confirms it. . . . Care practice can no longer be seen primarily as a matter of attending to physical needs, and no one can justify sentencing people with dementia to gross psychological neglect for three-quarters of every day. Even in this period of history, when cost-effectiveness has been made into a fetish, the warehouse model of residential care has become obscene."[4] He identifies the overarching psychological need of people with dementia as unconditional love.

Kitwood's views are taking hold. Indeed, transformational homes embrace them. As Judah Ronch writes in *Mental Wellness in Aging*, rather than focusing on the illness, competent caregivers increasingly focus on individuals, drawing on their past strengths and interests and helping them rally their defenses and coping skills. This not only is more effective than the pill approach, but also empowering and motivating for caregivers, according to Ronch.

Al Power, MD, assistant medical director of St. John's Home, an Eden Alternative home in Rochester, made a concerted effort to lower the use of antipsychotic medications among the residents he treats there. "Giving these drugs does not make them more comfortable, more happy, doesn't give them back control or dignity," he said. "All it does is sedate the behavior. They are quieter and have fewer episodes of combativeness—chloroform does that too!"

An article in *American Family Physician* discusses the long-time excessive use of antipsychotic drugs in nursing homes, "often solely for the convenience of staff."[5] The authors note that several studies found these drugs to be "no more effective than a placebo," with serious side effects.

Another study, published in the *New England Journal of Medicine*, followed 421 outpatients with Alzheimer's disease for 36 weeks to assess the effectiveness of these drugs. The researchers concluded that the adverse side effects offset the advantages of the drugs for the treatment of psychosis, aggression, or agitation in people with Alzheimer's disease. In many cases the drugs were little better than a placebo.[6] An editorial by Jason Karlawish, M.D., accompanying the article notes: "The Food and Drug Administration labels for antipsychotic medications state bluntly that they are not approved for the treatment of dementia-related psychosis, and they display a 'black box' warning: 'Elderly patients with dementia-related psychosis treated with atypical antipsychotic drugs are at an increased risk of death compared to placebo.' Yet clinicians, including me, continue to prescribe these drugs."[7]

Nationally, nearly 30 percent of nursing home residents are on antipsychotic medications, according to Dr. Power. The same was true at St. John's, before culture change. But today, just 5 percent of his patients are on antipsychotic medication, as the result of his shift to relationship-centered care.

Not only does Al Power believe the residents are better off, but also the cost savings is considerable. Some of the new antipsychotic drugs are quite costly—from one to four hundred dollars a month. Then there are the side effects, including rigid or uncontrollable movements, such as rocking back and forth, that can be "permanent and devastating," said Dr. Power, as well as increased risk of falls, fecal impaction, and decreased mobility. Recent studies also suggest an association of these drugs with strokes, faster cognitive decline, and even higher mortality. Because they cause sedation, the medications can contribute to bedsores. "For every dollar we spend on medications in nursing homes, we spend $1.33 on the side effects of the medications," Dr. Power said. "That's a big thing."

In a study in the *British Medical Journal*, researchers compared residents of twelve nursing homes in England: In half the homes, staff received training and support in person-centered care, including such skills as behavior management, awareness of environmental design, individualized interventions, active listening and communication, reminiscence techniques, and involvement of family caregivers. In the other six homes—the control group—residents with dementia continued to receive traditional medical care. After twelve months, 23 percent of residents in the intervention group were taking antipsychotic drugs compared to 42 percent of those in the control group. Behavior did not worsen when the drugs were eliminated.[8]

Looking at persons as individuals, identifying their strengths, and taking care of other physical problems can help reduce the challenging behavior associated with dementia. In 2005, the Alzheimer's Association launched a Quality Care Campaign to help long-term care providers target their efforts to improve dementia care. The campaign, developed in consultation with national experts, offers practical suggestions in four areas: nutrition, hydration, pain management, and social engagement. "People felt if you could deal with residents' hunger and thirst, pain, and boredom in an effective manner, a lot of the behavioral symptoms like agitation and depression could be mitigated," said Jane Tilly, a doctor of public health and the director of Quality Care advocacy. "If someone has an arthritic shoulder and can't express their pain other than resisting when someone is getting them dressed, then they get labeled as having difficult behavior."

The goal, said Tilly, is to encourage person-centered care. "We have some solid recommendations, backed by a variety of evidence—not just research, but practical, experiential evidence," she said. "So the value of the recommendations is they are very specific and meet special needs. They are also very consistent with culture change."

From my observations, person-centered care and a homey environment reduced the upsetting behavior of people with dementia that I often witnessed at traditional homes. The atmosphere was more peaceful in transformative homes. Tupelo's first Green Houses, for example, had many residents with severe dementia, yet I did not hear anyone cry out or appear agitated—or sedated, for that matter. This contrasted with many of the traditional nursing homes I visited, where the cries of people with dementia seemed to be accepted as normal.

"People with dementia are whatever the environment communicates to them," said David Green, former administrator of Evergreen in Oshkosh. "If they look at the environment and say, I don't belong here, they try to leave." In contrast, he said, if the environment looks like home, they will more likely offer to set the table than try to escape.

To keep their loved ones in a homier environment and to save money, many families move them to small board-and-care homes, at least for the early to mid stages of Alzheimer's disease. These are homes where the owner takes in a few people, providing room, board, some personal assistance, and companionship. Along with assisted living, board-and-care homes are an important piece of the long-term care mosaic.

The power of a home environment to transform behavior was a common theme among those I spoke with at nursing homes that had done away with the hospital model. Linda Bump at Bigfork, for example, said, "The residents who were severely impaired with their dementia and their social functioning in the big nursing home moved into that new environment, and their behaviors just went away. It looked normal. It felt normal. Their behaviors were fine—I'm talking about people through the years who had aggressive behaviors."

It's not only the homey setting. If that were the case, the difficult behavior would not occur in the person's own home. Researchers suggest that the physical environment of a nursing home or assisted living, while important, is only one component in transforming behavior. For residents to feel a sense of home, they must also be able to exercise independence and autonomy. "A nursing facility with a homelike décor that is operated with a rigid time schedule for rising and retiring, blocking of residents' schedules so they are always together in large groups, and staff-determined bathing schedules may be particularly difficult for the cognitively impaired person to understand and cope with," note researchers Margaret Calkins and Paul Chafetz.[9]

In a study that looked at environmental features of dementia-care units, researchers found "reduced aggressive and agitated behavior and fewer psychological problems" when residents had private, personalized bedrooms and surroundings that were simple to understand and negotiate. Having a variety of common areas and camouflaged exit doors also helped reduce depression, social withdrawal, misidentification, and hallucinations. The study concluded that dementia-care units "should strive to model their interior environments after homelike settings to reduce aggressive and other symptoms."[10]

Others say that the relationship between staff and residents is at least as important as the noninstitutional environment. "We overemphasize the importance of the physical attributes of the environment and under-appreciate the person attributes of the environment," said Peter V. Rabins, MD of Johns Hopkins University, coauthor of *The 36-Hour Day*. "If you can increase activities, if you can have staff that have more time to spend with individuals, that's much more important than how pretty the facility looks."

Who Is in There?

How do you know if someone with dementia is having a good life? What makes for a happy day, to people who have difficulty using language or even remembering what they did that morning? "It's a challenge in dementia," said Dr. Rabins. "Quality of life varies greatly. With severe memory impairment, they don't know what they've been doing the last day or two. We go by their behavior. Are they smiling? Do they look comfortable? Are they busy and active? We can use those things to measure quality of life."

Communicating with someone whose memories and language are vanishing is a formidable challenge. One of the disconcerting aspects of dementia is that the person may appear healthy and normal, until the late stage. I have carried on conversations with people for several minutes who I thought were cognitively intact, only to have them make a comment that revealed something was askew. In one case, "Mary Ann" and I had leisurely walked around the beautiful grounds of Oatfield Estates, where people are not segregated by their cognitive abilities. Mary Ann was a charming companion, sharing my interest in observing a large turtle in a pond and gazing at snowcapped Mount Hood in the distance. Over lunch, I asked how many children she had. For the first time, she looked uneasy. "Oh, I don't know," she said. "Several."

I have learned that asking people with dementia specific questions about their past can be embarrassing for both of us. Focusing on the present is much more comfortable—thus the importance of a rich environment.

Later I fell into easy conversation with "Lee," one of Mary Ann's housemates. Lee was an amiable man, friendly and articulate. He told me of his life, including such startling stories as his ninety-eight-year-old father still working as a cab driver. Lee said he himself ran a thriving therapy practice, and he was only in assisted living "on a temporary basis." Only after he began repeating himself, with details slightly changed—during the conversation he told me at various times he'd been working forty, thirty-five, and twenty-five years—did I realize I had no idea what was true in his stories. But his message was poignant and clear. "As a physical therapist, I worked in nursing homes," he said. "It was hard not being able to communicate well with people. I finally decided what those people need most is love. I would tell my employees who went to see clients in nursing homes that they should treat them like their own parent or grandparent and to remember they were once just like you or I. That same person is still inside."

The staff who work with people with dementia become adept at listening, interpreting, and honoring those whose conversation might baffle most of us. They discover activities that have meaning for residents, such as helping around the household, running errands, creating a piece of art, or caring for a pet. "I spend a lot of my time going into their reality," said Shari Brown, who worked in the household for people with dementia at Meadowlark Hills. "Someone may repeat something over and over and over. I answer her kindly and sweetly. She's losing her social skills, but what she has left, she wants to use. I love her for that. One woman recognized it was spring. The days are getting longer. She knew it was time to get the chicks."

Shari introduced me to "Warren," a man about my age, a college professor, with rapidly developing Alzheimer's. When she invited him to have a cup of coffee with us, he immediately tried to sit in thin air, in an invisible chair. Shari gently guided him to a table, where we all sat down. She brought him a coffee cup with a lid, which he could handle on his own. He had a gentle smile, and he listened to our conversation, although he was unable to contribute. He and Shari used to ride bicycles together, she told me.

Throughout our conversation, Shari referred to the residents as "my friends," as in, "Some of my friends here sleep longer or have different sleep patterns. If someone is up until two o'clock AM, they need to sleep longer in the morning." Her simple reference to "friends" said a lot about how she relates to people there.

"Above all, it's the relationships, not just with the elders, but with family members utmost," she said. "Success in those relationships drives a household. "

As Shari demonstrated, care for people with dementia has come a long way. Not too long ago, frustrated families and staff tried to convince people with dementia how irrationally they were behaving. If eighty-five-year-old Harry was looking for his mother, they would say, "Why, you know your mother has been dead for twenty years." This would upset Harry even more. "Why didn't anyone tell me? I would have gone to the funeral."

Instead, Shari explained, you must master the art of "redirection," by distracting—or humoring—the person. She told me of a man who became very agitated when a thunderstorm blew in. He said he must go get his cows back to the barn.

Rather than tell him he no longer had his farm and had sold his cattle long ago, Shari asked, "How many head of cows do you have?"

He told her how many, and she said, "Oh, you must have a hired hand to help out."

Yes, he did.

Shari assured him the hired hand would round up the cows, and the man calmed down.

At the Mount, Brenda Jennings is equally creative in connecting with people whose language is nearly gone. She asks herself, "What's inside this person? What can we do to make that present for them now?" She went on to give an example. "At Christmas, a woman I didn't know had a voice led others in carols half the night. How do you find that relationship, if you're used to connecting with words?"

Dr. Power relates an encounter between a resident at St. John's Home and Joanne Rader, a founder of the Pioneer Network and a nursing leader in compassionate dementia care. "Joanne was walking through the hallways and there was someone yelling, 'Mother, Mother,' over and over," he said. "Joanne put her hand on the woman's shoulder, and said, 'I'm right here, dear.' You can call it dishonest, I suppose, but the woman was expressing a need. Joanne was able to validate that and provide comfort."

In her practical guide *Learning to Speak Alzheimer's*, Joanne Koenig Coste describes the approach she developed and applied first to her husband, then in her work as a restorative aide in a nursing home. Her five-point "habilitative" program—make the physical environment work, know that communication remains possible, focus only on remaining skills, live in the patient's world, and enrich the patient's life—equally describes the strategies transformative homes use for all residents. Coste found that nursing home residents with whom she worked did "much better cognitively than they had done before and were participating more fully in daily living activities, such as dressing and bathing. All of the patients appeared calmer, which meant that their medications could be reduced. In this unit, restraints were removed; hugs were instituted."[11]

Creating an environment that welcomes family members, as discussed in the last chapter, is especially important for people with dementia, who cannot clearly communicate their needs. Families can help decorate residents' rooms with personal photos and heirlooms, take residents out to see old friends and relatives, and share residents' life stories with the staff. As a person's dementia worsens, the role of family members shifts, one article suggests, to one of "deliberate comforting. . . . This role was demonstrated by sitting with the older adults, talking with them, holding hands, listening to them, and attempting to reestablish or reaffirm connections to persons and places."[12]

Sue Matlock, whose father-in-law moved to the Mount because of dementia, said she had bonded with him in a new way once he was settled there. "I enjoyed knowing him at this time in his life," she said. "He had always been dogmatic. He softened, maybe because his world had shrunk."

His problems were serious, nonetheless. He behaved with suspicion toward his wife, Sue's mother-in-law, who lived on a different floor. "He thought she was unfaithful. He couldn't understand why they couldn't live together," she said.

I asked Sue and her husband, Bob, what constituted a good day for his father. "Being emotionally happy without pain was a good day," he said.

"To go for a walk," Sue said.

He enjoyed playing the violin at the Mount, and he loved to eat. "Both Mom and Dad loved playing horseshoes," said Sue. "The camaraderie with those residents was heartwarming—they supported each other. When they do a good job, they're really happy for each other. There were very touching experiences."

Appreciating ephemeral pleasures seems to lie at the heart of being with people with dementia. As many seasoned caregivers explain, if you can no longer remember the past or imagine the future, your life exists only in the here and now. "It's a life of moment-to-moment satisfaction and turning those moments into wonderful days," said Arbor Place codirector Dr. Fanburg. "That's one thing Alzheimer's teaches us—living moment to moment. Our goal is to help them live those moments comfortably and happily."

His wife, Eileen, added, "Joking isn't in the medical literature, but it gets a response."

Dancing, laughter, warm relationships—hard things to measure, but who would argue they are not fundamental, no matter what our condition might be?

Once again, the crucial importance of having a stable workforce is obvious. "Very high rates of staff turnover are bad for everybody—the person with the disease; the worker, who most likely is dissatisfied; people who run the facilities, because it's a challenge to keep them adequately staffed; and the quality of care, because the experience that one learns over time is a positive," said Dr. Rabins. "If people aren't staying in the job, not only does that mean they're dissatisfied, but it means the workforce is inexperienced, and they're always going to be undertrained."

What's So Special?

In recent years, retirement communities and nursing homes have begun advertising "special care units," a euphemism for dementia care. Whether people do better when they live exclusively with others who have dementia is unclear, according to Dr. Rabins. Part of the problem is that "special care" is ill defined and in far too many cases simply means a locked unit rather than highly skilled staff.

Transformative homes differ about whether people with dementia do better in their own "special" household or neighborhood or integrated with those who do not have cognitive impairment. Certainly those who are cognitively intact would prefer that those with dementia live elsewhere.

But some homes believe in a culture of inclusion. Kendal at Oberlin uses neither restraints nor a locked unit for people with dementia. In addition to the staff looking out for people's safety, other members of the community are expected to take responsibility if they see someone wandering off and to lend a friendly hand to help them find their way. During orientation, newcomers are told that a confused resident may invite herself to dine with them.

When I visited Kendal, I noticed a woman in the lobby who clearly had dementia. She sat in a chair, hugging a stuffed bear and looking worriedly at the front door. As residents came by to pick up their mail, they spoke kindly and reassuringly to her. Eventually, her husband came through the door, and she looked relieved. Together they strolled off. I realized that in many retirement communities, this woman would not be welcome to sit in the lobby, but would be shunted off in a locked wing.

The freedom to move about benefits not only those who are confused and forgetful, but also those who are still healthy. Independent residents know if they decline, they will not be banished to a separate wing, said Kendal administrator Barbara Thomas. One woman even said that Kendal's inclusive culture had removed her fear about becoming a widow. "She was no longer fearing the death of her spouse—what a gift!" said Barbara.

As part of its cultural transformation, the Mount also decided to do away with its dementia unit. Brenda Jennings explained how they went about the process of integrating their nursing home population:

We thought we were doing it very well when we had them separated. When we decided to change, one of the most difficult things was over-

coming fear on both sides. Those in a dementia-free world were not
thrilled to have "those people" around. Staff and families were up in arms.
The staff who took care of the dementia folks wanted to protect "their"
people. But the decision was made as part of wanting to be a community.
We used to split people up according to care needs—we'd given that up.
Aging in place means just because you walk through the door with all
your marbles doesn't mean you'll leave with them. All it takes is one TIA
[transient ischemic attack, or ministroke] to put you in a different reality
and then you're scooped up and moved. It just didn't feel right.

While we were doing the physical remodeling, we let the locked unit
downsize through attrition. We then spread people out in the neighborhoods. We tried to match people in ways that made sense. The reactions
of other residents ranged from fear to outrage. There were three ladies—
guardians of the hallways—that you had to run the gauntlet to get by.
Their mission in life was to be critical. There was some fear that people
would wander into the wrong room, and that happens some.

After the move, Brenda said, many of those with Alzheimer's seemed
to do better. "Some of the anxiety subsided, just to be in a more normal
environment," she said. "It's also easier for the staff to redirect the one or
two who need help. As our community has evolved over time, those who are
more alert and have more physical abilities are more protective of those with
dementia."

Challenges continue, though. One woman with Alzheimer's is particularly
difficult and gets angry if she is told she is in the wrong place. The staff is
learning that she enjoys helping around the neighborhood—she is willing
to help dust or fold laundry. The woman had also traveled all her life, "so
if someone needs to do an errand, they take her along," Brenda explained.
"Over time, people have become more tolerant of her."

I asked Brenda why I never heard anyone yelling, as I had in many other
nursing homes. "We don't find it acceptable to have yelling as a baseline
behavior," she said.

I have a lady who would get wound up—we had to figure out. What is it?
Is it internally a problem, or is it in the environment that is setting this
off? It may take a while, but we generally figure it out. You really focus on
that whole person, not just medical issues. It may be a very complex mental disorder, and we may have to manage it with meds. We had a woman
with terrible fear. Talk therapy was not an option for her. The other thing
that makes a big difference is staff relationships. Even in advanced dementias, they can't name you, but you're a familiar presence, touch, and

caring, and that's very comforting. Staff develop such strong attachments, and it really shows in how folks respond.

Hipp Tiniacos, who works in another neighborhood at the Mount, finds meaning in his relationships with people with dementia. "In the back of the brain, they listen, they know I'm there," he said. "It takes a lot of patience, a lot of understanding to make them feel they are safe with me. It's a simple matter—you begin with a lot of compassion."

He described how he treats those with dementia. "There is separation, but no border or frontier between me and them," he said. "Whatever the condition, you treat them with respect and as if there is no disorientation in their lives. There is no other way. There is one moment when the light comes into them—because they are human—and a little something opens, when you are close to them. Compassion and patience—with those two things, you can see a lot of beautiful things."

Chapter 11

"My Bags Are Packed"
Dying in the Nursing Home

> I have no time to speak to the residents. They cling to you.
> One resident called me in one night. She grabbed my arm
> and asked me to hold her. I gently removed her hand and
> explained that I had 16 residents to care for and could not
> stay. She died the next day. All she wanted was someone to
> be with her. I felt terrible.
> > —Nurse's aide, quoted in "What Makes for a Good
> > Working Condition for Nursing Home Staff?"

> The moment when they are leaving—the last moment
> of their life—that is hard. You are so close, and then one
> moment they have to go. And you have to be strong for
> them. Sometimes you are like their friend, or their son, or
> even the priest. I have said a blessing when no one else is
> around.
> > —Hipp Tiniacos, aide at the Mount

Perhaps no other aspect of life so starkly contrasts the old way and the new in nursing homes than dying. Unlike any other place where people live, death is an expected outcome of the nursing home experience. It may take several years for death to come, but people who are old, with complex medical problems, know that they are nearing the end of their lives. Today, in the United States, one in five deaths occurs in a nursing home. In addition, 30 percent of people who die in hospitals had been transferred there from nursing homes just a few days earlier. The number of people dying in nursing homes is expected to grow as hospitals continue to discharge all but the most acute patients. A Brown University study projected that by 2020, 40 percent of us will die in nursing homes. Yet rather than creating meaningful end-of-life care, nursing homes, in true medical model fashion, continue to treat death as a failure, an unwanted guest that is best left ignored. As one researcher notes, "In spite of serving as the setting for so many deaths, nursing homes are not prepared to care for the dying."[1]

Since the hospice movement began in the 1970s, we have learned a lot about what makes for a "good" death. Surveys consistently show that people want to die at home with loved ones around, and not in pain. But only about one-quarter of us die at home, and far too many of us die alone and in pain.

Many who die in pain are in nursing homes, where we would expect them to receive good medical care, at the very least. But nursing home residents in general, not only those who are dying, have significant untreated pain—from 30 to 80 percent of residents suffer needlessly, according to studies.[2] Pain goes untreated for many reasons: people with cognitive impairment may not be able to articulate their pain, older people may be stoic and not want to complain or bother harried staff, and pain is not taken seriously in older people in general, according to numerous studies.

Hospice nurses are experts at pain management and palliative, or comfort, care. All nursing home residents who are on Medicare have a hospice benefit, but only 1 percent of them take advantage of it.[3]

Why do nursing homes deal with death so poorly? Certainly it is not because of staff indifference. But researchers have found that nursing home staff, as well as family members, often have difficulty accepting death as a natural outcome. Sandra H. Johnson notes that the regulatory system also inadvertently creates incentives to promote a "death-denying culture within the nursing home."[4] Surveyors look askance at physical changes in residents, such as weight loss or dehydration, that are often a normal part of dying. To avoid being judged as giving poor care, nursing homes may inappropriately encourage tube feeding of residents, which prolongs death rather than saving life—a fine distinction to be sure, but one that is important to understand in order to give good end-of-life care.

"What if a proud and peaceful death here was a crowning achievement rather than a failure of medicine?" wonders Tom Gass in *Nobody's Home*. "We hide death as if we are ashamed of it: 'Lost another one.' When a resident dies here, we lock down the hall and hide the news and the body from fellow residents, as if they were unable to handle the one reality that clearly permeates these halls."

Ira Byock, MD, a pioneer in compassionate care of the dying, describes in his book *Dying Well: Peace and Possibilities at the End of Life* the fate of so many frail elders: "Passings that should have been peaceful turned gruesome. Nursing homes, for instance, routinely sent patients only moments away from death to the hospital by ambulance, lights and sirens blazing. By transferring the almost-dead to the emergency room, nursing homes could claim a mortality rate of nearly zero, while providing evidence to families, and any interested attorneys, that 'everything possible' had been done. This bizarre scenario extended not only to sudden deaths but also to people who were unconscious, in the final minutes of dying, and expected to die."[5]

Another kind of pain—that of spiritual emptiness and loneliness—also awaits dying nursing home residents. Perhaps they have no family members left, or family who live too far away to arrive in time. Unless a nursing home intentionally devotes staff or volunteers to sit with a dying person, she may die alone.

Once again, the pressing problems of understaffing and staff turnover get in the way. Add to this the fact that today's residents often arrive sicker and closer to death than people did in the past, so the time for staff to get to know them is condensed. "Now we find at least a third of our residents are going to live less than six months, another third less than two years," said Dr. Al Power of St. John's Home. "Only about a quarter of our long-term care residents are going to live for years. We're doing more palliative and end-of-life care than nursing homes used to do."

Yet the institution treats death as just one more series of unpleasant tasks: shield the roommate, dispose of the body, bag up the belongings, clean the room, get ready for the next victim, who will fill the bed as soon as possible because an empty bed means lost revenue. What does this say to the other residents about their fate? "If you think nobody sees that, you're dead wrong," said Meadowlark Hills' Steve Shields. "And if you don't think they personalize that—'Gosh, that's how I'm going to go'—you're dead wrong."

In fact, no one is satisfied with the way of dying in most nursing homes—not the dying person, not other residents, not the staff, not consulting hospice agencies, not physicians, and not bereaved family members. More than thirty years after the hospice movement was launched in the United States, a study in the journal *Geriatric Nursing* summed up the state of end-of-life care in today's nursing home: "Advance care planning is inadequate, discussions about life-sustaining treatment are rare, pain management is grossly inadequate, psychosocial support for families is lacking, and grief and bereavement services for families are limited."[6] We can add to this list, no grief support for staff.

Providing grief support to family members and staff, which costs little, can be deeply meaningful. In one study of a bereavement-support intervention, almost all support for families came from aides. Nursing homes were urged to designate staff members as bereavement leaders, ensuring that at least one be available at all times. These leaders would help families understand end-of-life care and would listen to family members. They would follow up after a death, extending sympathy to family members. They would also be responsible for holding periodic memorial services for those who had died in the nursing home.[7]

By most accounts, staff would welcome the opportunity to give their residents a better send-off. A survey of nursing home nurses, administrators, aides, and other staff by Sheryl Zimmerman and her colleagues at the University of North Carolina revealed how dissatisfied they were with the way death was handled. The most important change staff wanted was more time for aides to spend with people who are dying; next in importance were more use of volunteers, more staff education, staff available twenty-four hours, dying residents having a private room, more social worker time, counseling for staff on dealing with death, having a psychologist or chaplain on staff, obtaining preferences from residents about end-of-life care, involving hospice, and, to a lesser extent, encouraging staff to attend memorial services. With some differences in ranking, staff in assisted living and residential settings raised similar issues.[8]

In another study, a "Palliative Care Quiz" given to long-term care nurses confirmed that they, as well as physicians and aides, needed and wanted more education on giving good end-of-life care. The nurses flunked the quiz, with a mean score of twelve out of a possible twenty, or 62 percent. The study noted that plenty of resources were available to erase this knowledge gap, but nursing homes apparently were not making these resources available to their staff. Perhaps they didn't want to waste their money: The study noted that "rapid staff turnover often found in these long-term care facilities means that only limited benefit will accrue from in-service education."[9]

Other surveys confirm what aides have told me in interviews: Dealing with death is the most difficult part of their job. Some people may find this surprising, with the long litany of tough challenges aides face every day. I asked Hipp, at the Mount, if he could change anything about his job, what it would be. He thought a moment and said, "If I could change anything, I would talk to God about how to make these people live longer. And not to suffer."

A Tale of Two Mothers

"Connie" had a sadly typical experience when her mother died in a nursing home. Connie was a long-distance family caregiver who lived in Washington, D.C., while her mother, who had Alzheimer's disease, lived in California in a nursing home—the best that money could buy. Three thousand miles away, Connie depended on the staff to let her know when problems arose. This grew ever more important as her mother's dementia worsened, and she could not communicate directly with her daughter about her medical condition. Yet she was a survivor. She fell frequently, breaking multiple bones, but she managed to keep on going. Because of her mother's resilience, Connie was unprepared for the end.

Just before Christmas, her mother broke her hip, and her condition rapidly worsened. Connie suggested hospice but was assured by the nursing home staff that her mother was stable. "As she got weaker, nobody ever said to me, 'She's dying,' or helped me to know that," she said.

Connie went to visit the following week. She realized the end could not be too far away. Sooner than anyone expected, her mother died—sadly, at a time Connie was not present in the nursing home. When she got the call, she rushed there. No staff member was on hand to greet or support her. She felt terribly alone. "No one from the nursing home was there. No one was saying anything to me. She had lived there for nine years," Connie said in disbelief.

Mourning rituals are part of all human communities—why not the nursing home? To Connie, the absence of any acknowledgment of her mother's death was deeply painful. Her mother had the misfortune to die on a weekend. "It was only afterwards that I wondered, What was it like for staff members who were there on Friday and came on Monday and she was dead and gone?" Connie said. "Or for other people in that facility—she was very active. Couldn't they have some ritual to celebrate the life? There was absolutely nothing. I wonder how a nursing home does that."

To make matters worse, she had been assured that her mother's room would be left as it was for a few days, allowing her time to pack up her mother's belongings. But when she got there the next day, "someone was in her room, and all of her belongings were in these four garbage bags. It was horrible. The nursing home cost ten thousand dollars a month out of pocket. It was unbelievable."

Sadly, Connie's experience is not unusual, down to the black plastic garbage bags that symbolize to many family members what their loved one is worth to the nursing home.

Contrast this experience with that of Rose Marie Fagan. As mentioned, Rose Marie, of the Pioneer Network, was a family caregiver to her mother, who lived at Fairport Baptist nursing home.

My mother died on my birthday. I came to believe she chose that day, and I'm very honored. We went to visit her that morning. Every year I'd call her on my birthday and say thanks for having me. We'd laugh every year. That morning I went to see her, and I could tell right away she'd taken a turn. She had congestive heart failure and congestive renal failure, and she was filling up with fluid. We could put her in a hospital, but we all agreed to let nature take its course. We called the family in. The priest did last rites. My mother talked to my sister on the phone in California. All those things were taken care of. She died when we were there. They let us stay as long as we wanted and included us in everything.

After she died, they rang a chime three times over the intercom system and said her name. Staff from all over the house and residents came in to her room. We did a bedside memorial service with some prayers. Then, what I loved, the residents and staff shared their reminiscences and stories of my mother. Then we shared with them, what it meant for us for her to be there in community—how grateful we were to the staff to have my mother gain enough function and strength to enjoy our last two holidays with her. One by one, after that, the staff and residents went to my mother and said good-bye, just like at a funeral home. We covered her with a hand-embroidered cover. Then there was a procession of staff, residents, and family members—instead of the nursing home taking her body to the basement to a loading dock. We went out to a hearse, and it was so beautiful. They let us remove her things when we were ready. It was dignified. My mother was a very dignified person, and there was a peace to the whole thing. Can you imagine for staff, how much more meaningful their work is when they can really be in relationship with the residents and help them have a meaningful life?

A Better Way to Die

Dying wasn't always such a meaningful experience at Fairport Baptist. The scene Rose Marie describes is rooted in a culture based on relationship and respect. As administrator Garth Brokaw explains, as part of the process of changing the nursing home's culture, the staff developed a statement of Fairport Baptist's core values. The last of these reads: "We believe in the sanctity of life and the sacredness of death." The staff recognized that the standard way of doing things—whisking the body away, concealing it on the way down to the basement and the loading dock, putting the belongings in the black trash bags—in no way honored the sacredness of death. "So we said, if you come in the front door of the Baptist home, maybe you should go out the front door of the Baptist home," said Garth. He credits front-line caregivers with coming up with the ritual of ringing the chime and saying the person's name, so that anyone in the building who knew the deceased could gather. A simple ceremony was written up, and any staff member is empowered to read it at the bedside.

During my visits to the Mount, I was impressed by the seriousness of purpose with which the staff cared for those at the end of life. I was invited to attend a meeting between nurses and social workers and their counterparts at a hospice agency the Mount employed. They discussed the challenge of integrating hospice-care plans with nursing-care plans and planned how to work better as one team to serve those at the end of life. Two dozen people spoke in earnest for an hour or more. At the end, administrator Charlene Boyd reviewed what each had agreed to do to move forward.

"What a joy it is to work with Providence Mount Saint Vincent!" the hospice social worker said. And what a contrast to studies in which hospice agency nurses give low marks to nursing homes.

The most tender stories I heard from staff related to the deaths of cherished residents. "Old people are at peace and ready to die," said Lyn Frisch, a nurse and neighborhood coordinator at the Mount. "One man told me, 'My bags are packed and I'm waiting for the good Lord to come get me.'"

I thought of my friend Lynne, whose mother has some dementia and lives in a nursing home in Kansas. Lynne asked her if she knew how old she'd be on her next birthday.

"No, I don't believe I do," she said.

Lynne told her she would be ninety-five years old. Without missing a beat, her mother replied, "Uh-oh, time to go!"

Lynne's sister, Anne, asked her, "Well, Mom, where are you going?"

She said with a twinkle in her eye, "Well now, that's not up to me, is it?"

This acceptance of what lies ahead is part of the wisdom of growing very old.

Another aide at the Mount, Marsha Wilson, said her work with elders had helped her overcome panic attacks about her own death. "It makes me feel easier about when I have to die," she said. "You talk and they're ready to die, and they're not scared."

Mount aide Hipp Tiniacos believed that dying sometimes brought an intense awareness to people who had long had dementia. "People who haven't spoken for years will open as they are dying. A resident had a relative far away from here. She was feeling unhappy about that. At the moment the resident was close to leaving us, I said, 'God bless you.' She said, 'Thank you for being there, and I will look for you after. You connected me with the people I love.' I think I gave her peace. You have many memories like that."

At Wesley Village, staff created a Moment of Peace basket with relaxation tapes, prayers, aromatherapy supplies, and music for people who are dying. When a resident begins getting hospice care, an angel is put on the door to let the dietary staff know to bring extra meals for family members who are staying. Rev. Jim Stinson holds memorial services especially for staff to honor every resident who dies. Family members are invited.

I share a scripture or inspirational poem and move on to them telling stories. How did they really feel about caring for this person? How much of a strain was it to be loving and kind? What kind of gifts did they bring to that person? I try to be honest. It gives both the family and staff permission to say what they're really feeling, rather than just trying to be nice. Staff need to work through that feeling. Otherwise they're really not remembering the person and not doing honor to the person or to themselves. At first, people said, "Do we really want to do this?" And now if I don't do it right away, staff call me and ask.

Gary Kornblith recalled with pleasure the memorial service held for his mother at Kendal at Oberlin.

Rather than do a typical memorial service, we did a celebration, complete with the jazz combo from the conservatory. We did it as an event we thought she would enjoy. Everybody turned out—some of the folks from one of the restaurants she used to go to, her hairdresser came from the mall. I got letters from people in town, storekeepers who enjoyed having her as a customer, the head of the local artists' association. One always wonders, Did I do enough? But my sense is she really had enjoyed most of the last ten years and had not felt she was just waiting to die. She had really had a chance to do things she hadn't done before. She got to live in a tight-knit community and be a star.

Families frequently choose to hold memorial services at these homes, recognizing that it was these relationships that gave their loved one meaning in the final years. Perhaps this is the true test of transformation—that families would choose the nursing home as the sacred space to celebrate and honor a life.

Steve Shields was especially moved by the death of Betty, a resident of the household at Meadowlark called Lyle House. As he tells the story,

Betty couldn't speak and she was in a wheelchair, but she spoke volumes with her eyes. And everybody loved Betty. They have never heard Betty speak. But you find different ways of listening. The beauty of [transforming the culture] is that relationships grow. And they flourish and the residents create solidarity among their house. Like we have solidarity in our homes. It happens. It really happens.

Well, Betty began to actively die in her room. And the dynamic of that process really spoke to this vision. When Betty began to die, the staff began to vigil. This wasn't policy. It wasn't procedure, it wasn't planned. It was a spontaneous expression of humanity. And so they vigiled Betty. And her family began to vigil Betty. And when Betty died, that was the most intimate connection between Betty and, I believe, God and this family that were blood children and grandchildren and great-grandchildren and Lyle House family. It became interconnected and intertwined. I went to Betty's funeral—we went to the same church. It was a beautiful service. And then after the service, they had a second service, and they had it at Lyle House in the living room. And you know what? Family members of other residents who had already died came back to Lyle House. And they brought covered dishes. And that wasn't organized. It was what you do. It was an organic household thing.

The most beautiful thing about that service was that residents shared their feelings about Betty. One woman who couldn't speak very much said, "I loved Betty." And the staff shared. So it was an old-time, in-the-parlor service born out of our decision to make home. When her daughter stood up at the last, she gave a beautiful elegy and said, "Our biggest wish for Mother was that she would die at home. And she did."

PART III

Making the Case for Change

Fundamental change begins in the human
heart. If we really don't believe that people
are still people because they have a dementia,
we will not care for them as persons, but
as objects of medical maintenance. If we
really don't believe that elderhood can be
a great age of enlightenment and societal
participation, then we will continue to relate
to elders as retirees on the golf course. Each
of us must work deeply on our own journey of
aging, transforming our traditional fears and
uncertainties into a hopeful, joyful embrace of
who we are and our new capacities for growth
and giving.

— Bill Keane, long-time culture change
leader

Chapter 12

Too Good to Be True?
Overcoming Obstacles

To change a culture is never easy. It not only involves a
challenge to privilege and power, but also the dismantling of
deep psychological resistance.

—Tom Kitwood, *Dementia Reconsidered*

Unless the culture changes, too many residents fall by the
wayside. We may have the knowledge, but, apparently,
the will is too often lacking. Change is never easy! Change
toward a new orientation cannot be imposed but rather must
come from within.

—Sheldon S. Tobin, "The Historical Context of
'Humanistic' Culture Change in Long-Term Care"

Bill Thomas is fond of saying that transforming nursing homes is akin to
coaxing the draft horses on his farm to work in tandem. He told me
this as I was bouncing along on a wooden wagon seat behind two 1800-
pound horses, Ned and Dan, plodding past the family's wind turbine and
woodpile. "Only by working in partnership can you effect change," he said,
patting the horses. "If you try to force change, the status quo is too massive
and ingrained to budge."

I did not imagine myself in this pastoral pocket of New York when I set
out to learn about new ways older people might live. But the leaders of the
Pioneer Network turned out to be an eclectic bunch, scattered across the
country. Bill Thomas is both the best known of these leaders and the most
unusual, an unlikely mix of middle-aged hippie, Harvard-educated physician,
and jet-setting international speaker. In June 2006, *U.S. News and World
Report* named him one of "America's Best Leaders." More than one admin-

istrator has told me they were so inspired by hearing just one talk by Bill Thomas that they immediately started their nursing home on the culture-change journey.

What I have learned from him and others is that deep, transformative change is possible—but never easy. It requires making tough decisions, eliminating some jobs and reinventing others, throwing out schedules and rethinking rules, all while convincing skeptical staff that the old way of doing things—the way they've been taught through years of training and experience—is wrong. Some employees resign rather than change. Family members complain that too much freedom is dangerous for their loved ones. Regulators challenge the wisdom of giving residents more choice and thus perhaps less safety. Funds must be raised for renovations or training.

"Corporate cultures don't allow for a lot of flexibility, and this is not just in the for-profits, but big nonprofit chains as well," long-term care researcher Robyn Stone told me. "It makes it harder because you need a lot of flexibility when you're talking about organizational change, and that flies in the face of a lot of corporate culture—despite the fact that large corporations like Toyota and IBM were pioneers in culture change. There's no reason why it couldn't be done."

The reimbursement system is also skewed. Instead of being rewarded for wellness, nursing homes are rewarded for poor outcomes. Al Power of St. John's explained, "We get paid more if someone has a bedsore than if they don't. If we heal it, they pay less. If they are bedridden, and we get them to walk, we get paid less. That's the basic problem."

But beyond that issue—and beyond the scope of this book—we have no rational plan for paying for long-term care, especially when the baby boomers will need it. The current system of using Medicaid as a last resort clearly satisfies no one: Middle-class elders must impoverish themselves in order to have their nursing home expenses covered (or hire lawyers to help them conceal their assets, an ethically problematic solution); low-income people, whom Medicaid was meant to benefit, are increasingly shortchanged as funds are used for long-term care insurance for everyone; and providers must go hat in hand every year to the government to plead for higher reimbursement. Meanwhile, state budgets are stretched thin.

We need to create a rational, fair system that in its ideal form would encompass health care, affordable housing, transportation, and other needs of older people that today go unmet. As a first huge step, we need to figure out how to pay for the long-term care of the next generation. Perhaps we should mandate long-term care insurance, just as we require people to insure their homes and their automobiles. Others argue for a system of universal long-term care insurance to cover most expenses, with individuals paying premiums to the federal government. Whatever mix of public and private financing we develop, the nation would be wise to begin a serious conversation—now—about how to fund long-term care before the deluge of aging baby boomers needs services.

Beyond the reimbursement issues, the field of long-term care has an underlying cynicism about why fundamental change won't work. Among the refrains: "Regulators won't let us innovate"; "We can't afford it" (whatever it is); "We might get sued"; "Our residents are too sick to enjoy life anyway"; "Our staff is too transient to care." And besides, "culture change" is just a passing fad, so why bother?

The greatest barrier to transformation, though, is not a financial or regulatory one, but one of attitude or will. "Change," one nurse told me, when I asked what the biggest obstacle was. "Change. People hate change. People translate the idea [of giving residents] more choices as meaning more work. They also see change as a criticism and a threat."

This is not to make light of the very real challenges facing long-term care. But sticking to the old way of doing things will not address these problems. If anything, crises such as a labor shortage and an incoherent payment system should force providers and society as a whole to rethink the current system—or lack thereof.

Reflecting on all the challenges, Steve Shields explained why they were able to move forward at Meadowlark Hills: "The vision was painted so strongly and in front of everybody that it became holy. Truly. So that's how we endured all that. The mission and holiness of that vision was just supreme. It was absolutely supreme."

Viewing this movement as a moral, ethical imperative may sound too idealistic. But only by seeing the fate of elders through a moral lens will we be compelled to act for those most in need—those who not only are old, sick, frail, or forgetful but who also are too poor to pay for care. What is impressive about this movement is its commitment to all elders, including those who depend on Medicaid. Only by supporting universal access to a life with dignity, no matter our age, income, or frailty, they suggest, will we truly transform the culture of our society.

Until recently, no such vision existed. Instead, the goal has been merely to stop dreadful things from happening. This is fostered in part by the government survey process, which is long on finding fault and short on identifying success. Every twelve to fifteen months, state inspectors descend on every nursing home to uncover poor practices that pose harm to residents. Without their efforts, many nursing homes would undoubtedly be far worse than they are. Yet many administrators and staff feel they receive no reward for going the extra mile and providing exemplary care. "Absence of bedsores, absence of depression, absence of malnutrition—these are hardly evidence of a good quality of life or goals to inspire generations of care providers," observes researcher Rosalie Kane.[1]

While inspiration and passion may nudge some nursing home owners, others will be unconvinced—especially when the owners are corporate shareholders. They demand evidence that investing in change will yield a payoff in terms of eased regulation, lowered expenses, or increased revenue.

"Culture change in general has been slow to spread because no one has presented the empirical evidence that changing one's culture leads to better financial performance," said David Farrell of the Rhode Island Quality Improvement Organization. "All we've had is an inspirational message. No one was able to fill the gap—not only is it the right thing, but it makes perfect business and clinical sense." To address this need, Farrell developed a presentation that lays out the business case for culture change and has delivered it to providers and regulators in nearly every state.

Farrell draws clear links between having a stable workforce, reducing costs, and giving high-quality care:

> We're finding that we can now specifically pinpoint what leaders do in high-performing nursing homes, specific actions that they take that lead to culture change, higher quality, and better service. We're beginning to tap into that and to say to leaders, the evidence is really strong that if you don't involve staff in problem solving, if you don't reward and recognize staff, if you hole yourself up in your office as opposed to having the door open because you're always out with the staff—these are the actions that distinguish high-performing, low-turnover nursing homes. The evidence is mounting.

Why Transformation "Won't Work"— Debunking the Myths

"We can't afford it."

Most people associate high quality with high cost. But what is surprising is that transformative homes do not have to cost more to operate than traditional nursing homes. Many of the changes cost little. Fundamentally, the change is one of attitude. It requires reorganization and relationship building, rather than investment in fancy surroundings. Some of the very best nursing homes serve primarily people who are on Medicaid. From the outset, Steve McAlilly was determined that the Green Houses could be judged a success only if they were affordable, at a cost supported by Medicaid. Trace-way achieved this goal, as did many other transformative homes that serve primarily low- to moderate-income people.

"Culture change is ethically important," Mark Latham of Pleasant View said. "What makes me think it will be successful is that it goes hand-in-hand with smart business."

I asked him to lay out the business case as if he were trying to convince a colleague. "This business is so difficult that the only people who work in it are for the best interests of the customer," he said. "The employee wants to be in an environment that supports home and a person's values. If the employee is doing that, they're happy. Customer satisfaction rates go up, and employee satisfaction rates go up. That leads to higher employee retention and a stable workforce—which is much less expensive."

Reducing staff turnover and absenteeism may be the single strongest argument that reform advocates could make to convince hidebound nursing home operators. To keep staff positions filled is an enormous drain on the bottom line of most nursing homes. As discussed throughout this book, trans-formative homes make significant strides in stopping the costly hemorrhaging of staff. David Green, former administrator of Evergreen, cautioned, though, that the first year or two during a transition, turnover may actually *increase* as some employees refuse to embrace change. During this time of transi-tion, surveys also may reveal more problems than usual. At Evergreen, staff turnover was 18 percent in 1993, rose to 36 percent when culture change was introduced, but then settled down to between 11 and 16 percent and has stayed there.

After St. John's became an Eden Alternative home, Dr. Al Power said, they were able to stop using agency staff, saving $4 million a year. "It's had so many good results," he said. "Our surveys have been without a major deficiency, and our elder and family satisfaction has gone up every year." Di-rect-care staff turnover is down from more than 30 percent to 13 percent.

In a study examining cost, nursing researcher Marilyn Rantz concluded that high-quality care is actually *less* expensive to deliver than is low-qual-ity care. In what should by now be a familiar refrain, she found that higher staff retention led to increased efficiency and better-quality outcomes that in turn led to lower costs. The average cost per patient day was $13.50 less in high-quality homes, for an annual savings of $440,000 in a home with ninety residents.[2]

Money is simply not an obstacle to change, said Charlene Boyd, admin-istrator of the Mount. In fact, saving money on operating costs was one of the Mount's motivations to change. "It didn't cost more at all," she said of the nursing home's transformation in the early 1990s. "By reducing middle management and decentralizing services, we could then put more money in direct-care work." The Mount eliminated thirty-five middle-management positions through attrition, buyouts, and retirements. All floor staff were cross-trained in food service, laundry, housekeeping, and personal assistance. And the Mount, unlike many nursing homes, is unionized.

Food costs, too, go down when residents eat when they are hungry, rather than on the institution's schedule. The number of special diets is reduced to a few, as homes learn it is more important for elders to eat appetizing food than to have meals medicalized into inedible ordeals. This leads both to less food waste and to reduced use of dietary supplements, while at the same time residents maintain or even increase their weight.

Personalized care leads to a need for fewer antipsychotic medications and incontinence supplies, two other areas of significant savings.

With thousands of aging nursing homes around the country in need of updating, now is the time to invest in building renovations as well. Here too, smaller may be better. Constructing family-size homes, rather than huge institutions, is likely to be less expensive, depending on the cost of land, in part because fireproofing large buildings costs considerably more.

"We as an industry are trying to reinvent ourselves," said Charlene Boyd. "If we would look at how other businesses work, and how they have to change their models to survive and do business differently, that is what we need to do as well. The consumer, too, is demanding a different kind of service. They're demanding to have their rights restored, to have more normalcy, more community, all those kinds of things. If we're going to stay in this business, then those are the values and philosophies they want. Therefore let's figure out a way to do it."

Charlene raises the final reason why transformative homes should appeal to operators with an eye on the bottom line: Occupancy rates are high. Imagine that in your own community you could choose the Mount, Meadowlark Hills, or a Green House versus a traditional nursing home. Is there any question what you would choose?

"Don't tell me that you don't have the money to do it," said Karen Schoeneman of the Centers for Medicare and Medicaid Services (CMS). "I'm not buying it, and neither are the rest of the culture-change leaders."

"The regulators won't let us."

More than anything else, nursing home administrators hate regulations. They hate the voluminous paperwork, the annual surveys, the sense that regulators are out to get them. Surveyors can find fault with hundreds of items, large and small. Administrators argue that the punitive approach does little to encourage higher quality and in fact can be a barrier to innovation.

An example from Ridgewood illustrates the problem. A resident who had some dementia very much wanted an electric wheelchair. He lobbied every-one he could. The staff told him no, it wouldn't be safe. But he was insistent, and eventually they felt they had to let him try. Within the first week, he had two accidents with the chair. In the second one, he crashed into a wall and broke his leg. That was the end of the electric wheelchair for him.

"When the surveyor came, he wanted to cite us for giving a resident a lethal weapon," said administrator Bonnie Kisielewski.

Lethal weapon? A wheelchair?

"Yes, they said the electric wheelchair was a lethal weapon because it could be used to endanger himself or others."

During the following days, while the survey team was onsite, Bonnie patiently explained that theirs was a home that believed in resident rights. "We had to let [the resident] fail—that's his choice," she explained. "We were able to support that decision with our culture-change philosophy."

She must have been persuasive. When the final survey was in, the home had no citations.

Meadowlark Hills was not so lucky. A 2005 survey cited multiple deficien-cies, in part because the home allowed a resident to go outdoors alone when he wished to smoke a cigarette—not only that, it "allowed" him to have a cigarette lighter. "We knew this man should not be restricted," said Steve Shields. Rather than give in to the surveyors and limit the man's freedom, Meadowlark Hills had him undergo assessments by a psychiatrist, nurse, and occupational therapist, who all confirmed that going outdoors did not pose a risk for him. The state accepted that. But there was still the matter of the cigarette lighter. The man refused to give it up. The director of nursing ex-plained the problem to him, but the man insisted he was not going to allow his lighter to be taken away, and besides, he was not about to set anyone on fire. Finally, he came up with a compromise: He would sell his seventy-nine-cent lighter to the director of nursing for two dollars. The deal was struck. Meadowlark went so far as to rig up a lighter on the outside of the building so residents could light their cigarettes. "We were ready to go to the mat for this guy," said Steve.

Pam Elrod of Genesis blames regulations for just about everything that is wrong with nursing homes.

This is an industry of control, since its inception. The state and federal government expects you to control everything—about care, about the en-vironment, about safety. We're the most regulated industry in the world. It's all the federal government's fault. Now the pendulum has shifted because of public sentiment. They want more choice, and a more home-like environment, and all that is about *not* having control. The meteor has hit, and we're all still dinosaurs. We're still trying to do it the old way, even though the world is changing around us. You say you want residents' rights, but everything you measure is the opposite. We have to find new ways to measure what success means.

The problem, of course, is that regulations were not created by a gaggle of bureaucrats with nothing better to do. Karen Schoeneman of CMS tells administrators that if they truly believe a regulation is unreasonable, they should challenge it. "The regulations come from the public wanting something. It comes from public pressure, usually through Congress and then to us: Here's a problem, cover it with some regulation. Regulations change because the public wants them to, too."

In recent years, Karen has aggressively educated surveyors around the country, explaining that culture change embodies the Nursing Home Reform Law. "We're interested in surveyors understanding we believe in culture change," she said. "It implements our law. Our law says give [nursing home residents] the best they can have."

For all their griping, most nursing home administrators would probably acknowledge that they must be regulated. When pressed, most I spoke to agreed that the marked decline in the use of restraints would not have come about had it not been for regulations. "We're dealing with an extremely vulnerable customer base," said Mark Latham. "We should be closely regulated. But we're suffocating under regulation. You could have instead a survey team come in as a partner for improvement. There should be a level of trust and help from the government for struggling buildings, instead of not trusting and trying to catch them. Surveyors could share information with poor performers. We work better trying to measure quality rather than deficiencies. We need to get away from the punitive and work towards the cooperative and bring the low end up. You really don't have people who want to do a bad job."

Perhaps, but horror stories still show up regularly in the media. In April 2006, the National Citizens' Coalition for Nursing Home Reform issued a stomach-churning exposé, "The Faces of Neglect: Behind the Closed Doors of Nursing Homes," that documented still more shocking examples of neglect and abuse.

Those on the front end of transformation say that the antiregulation argument is overblown. They urge their colleagues to show a little backbone, be proactive, and shake off the hunker-down mentality. "I don't like deficiencies either, but after all these years, I'm not going to lie down and roll over if I can help it," said Garth Brokaw. "Some things are right, and some things are not right, and someone has to draw a line in the sand. I found that for the most part if you do it in a reasonable way, [regulators] are much better at listening than they used to be. There are some exceptions to that, but I don't live in fear of it anymore. So many times, decisions in nursing homes get made out of fear of a survey."

Steve Shields agrees. "I'm a believer in the fact we need regulations," he said. "We have to have a system that works for seventeen thousand nursing homes across the country—all these different providers with different ethics and different standards. I'm not in the camp that whines about regulations and regulators. The regulatory system, the survey and enforcement system, is broken, just like the industry is broken. If we stay on track to fix ourselves and make ourselves well, the enforcement will follow suit. It's going to take time."

At Traceway, Steve McAlilly met early on with state officials and surveyors as planning was underway for the nation's first Green Houses. "We found there's a myth about the regulations in the minds of both management and the regulators," he said. "The regulations have been interpreted differently than the letter of the law. Most regulations make sense—there may be a little overkill. The regulations are written for the lowest common denominator."

The best way to ease regulations or litigation is for nursing homes to improve quality of care and quality of life. Decades of doing things the old way, while leading to some improvements, have not brought the regulatory relief that everyone says they want.

"We'll get sued."

Rising liability costs are a big concern for all nursing homes. In one study, providers reported an annual average increase of $130,086, or 143 percent, between 2001 and 2002. Nursing home trade associations argue that an increase in lawsuits, including frivolous ones, drives steep rate increases. Consumer advocates such as NCCNHR argue that market forces, not litigious elders, push premiums up. In fact, there is little evidence that lawsuits are frivolous, according to Bernadette Wright of the AARP Public Policy Institute, who reviewed the literature on litigation.[3]

A study by California Advocates for Nursing Home Reform found that a small number of homes were repeat offenders. Ten percent of 577 facilities were responsible for 47 percent of the lawsuits, for example. "Victims of elder abuse should not be blamed for the alleged liability insurance crisis," the study concluded. "The best way for nursing homes to avoid lawsuits and liability is to improve care."[4]

No studies of transformative nursing homes have yet explored whether their new way of doing things has led to more litigation or to less. Certainly no administrator I interviewed identified litigation as a problem. Drawing on lessons learned from malpractice suits of physicians, one can infer that the stronger and more open the relationships among employees, administrators, residents, and family members, the less likely that a nursing home will be sued. A study in the *Western Journal of Medicine*, for example, found that physicians' poor communication skills put them more at risk of lawsuits than did their actually doing anything wrong.[5] "I do think reducing litigation is a possible byproduct of a culture-change type of environment, although it has not been documented," said David Stevenson of Harvard University, who researches the relationship between litigation and quality of care in nursing homes.

Steve Shields believes that during the transition from the old to the new, nursing homes may face an increased risk of litigation. "If it's a wholesale change, which is what we advocate, there is chaos in the beginning, until things stabilize," he said. "At all levels the risk is high during that first year, including the risk of litigation."

But that risk drops over time. "Inherently it's much more relational," he said, "and the residents and families are much more in control of what happens because they're intrinsically driving it. In the long run, overall, there is less litigation risk, just from a person-to-person, organization-to-customer standpoint." Meadowlark, he added, has not been sued.

Bonnie Kantor of Ohio State agrees. Transformative homes, she said, "now know what physicians know. The best way to keep lawsuits away is to have good relationships."

"But will it work?"

Steve Shields claims he once, in frustration, told a noted researcher that if she saw two dogs, one trapped in a tiny cage and the other free to run through the woods, she would insist on doing a study to analyze which dog was happier.

It may seem obvious that giving elders choice, warm relationships, and a pleasant home is better than confining them to hospital-like institutions. Nevertheless, nursing homes and many academics insist on rigorous research to demonstrate measurable improvements in residents' well-being.

Rose Marie Fagan, leader of the Pioneer Network, reflected on the role of research. "It is important—and it also seems stupid, like we have to do research to understand that if you treat people well, take care of your staff and give them opportunities for advancement, you might retain staff better." She laughed. "A researcher will say, it's not valid until it's studied. When I think of the zillions of dollars that go into research to prove what is obvious—but we need research to affect public policy, and it's part of the system."

One research challenge is that "culture change" and "transformational" are not clearly defined and are interpreted differently from home to home.

Thus comparing a "culture-change" home with a traditional institution is difficult. In standard research, you must control for variables. In this case, there are almost too many possible variables to consider—consistent staffing, a beautiful garden, enriching activities, a low-stress environment, and so on. And what are you comparing—resident satisfaction, clinical outcomes, staff retention?

"If you are saying you are a 'culture-change' home, we need to be able to see what exactly did you change —- your policies, your building, your staff enhancements," said Karen Schoeneman of CMS. To that end, she and consultant Carmen S. Bowman, owner of Edu-Catering—Catering Education for Compliance and Culture Change, created "Artifacts of Culture Change," a document that nursing homes are free to use. The self-assessment questionnaire identifies seventy-nine concrete changes, each afforded a certain number of points, that reflect a change from an institutional to a resident-directed model. The list ranges from having bathroom mirrors that are wheelchair accessible to having consistent assignments for staff, doing away with the nurse's station, and having regular interaction with children or pets. "This is a tool that a home can use to see where they're at, relative to their peers. They can see what they've accomplished, and they can get new ideas," said Karen. "Researchers can figure out who is in the culture-change group." They could then compare homes with very high scores with traditional homes on any variety of measures.

Although rigorous research of transformational homes is scarce, studies have compared discrete components of traditional versus transformational homes. For example, a study in the May 2006 *British Medical Journal* compared family-style dining with traditional nursing home meals, where food is served on a plastic tray in a dull environment. The study found that over a six-month period, not only did quality of life improve, as you might expect, but those eating family-style maintained both their weight and their ability to function, in contrast to those in the control group. Numerous studies discussed in this book have shown the benefits of consistent staffing, a hallmark of culture change and of high-quality care.

In addition, homes monitor their own progress. At Wesley Village, the Planetree model guides continuous quality improvement. Each year, staff on all levels, families, and residents evaluate progress on each of the Planetree components (see Appendix D) over the previous year and focus on goals for the coming year. Since Wesley Village implemented culture change, the number of residents throughout the campus who rated "overall quality of services" excellent increased from 75 to 94 percent from 2003 to 2004. In the nursing home the number of restraints decreased by 60 percent and the number of pressure sores dropped 45 percent.[6]

Studies of the Mount found significant improvements in many important areas. From 1995 to 2001, the average number of people with functional decline fell from 82 to 3, with range-of-motion problems from 33 to 5, with weight loss from 20 to 3, with bedsores from 11 to 2, and with restraints from 22 to 2.[7]

University of Minnesota researcher Rosalie Kane conducts ongoing studies of the Green Houses. The preliminary findings at Traceway were promising. In addition to the expected improvements in quality of life, she said, the medical indicators also looked good. Kane and her colleagues examined data from the Green Houses and compared them to data from the same period at Cedars, Traceway's traditional nursing home, and another nursing home owned by the same nonprofit. "There were no negative effects of being in the Green House," Kane said. "Some might have worried that without extensive health surveillance and supervision [of the shahbazim], you would see negative outcomes, but that was not the case. Any statistically significant differences favored the Green House." Specifically, people living in the Green House had less decline in their ability to perform "activities of daily living," a lower prevalence of depression, less incontinence without a toileting plan, and less use of antipsychotic drugs without a diagnosis.

"The Green House encourages functioning and helps people maintain functioning," she said. "The distances are smaller. People are watching to assist residents getting to the toilet, with eating, and to encourage people to eat. The food is good and fresh and visible, and that encourages feeding oneself."

Kane's findings regarding the staff were even more striking. Compared to the two control groups, the staff reported they felt more empowered to assist residents, knew residents better, experienced greater "intrinsic and extrinsic" job satisfaction, and were more likely to remain on the job.

On the other hand, a study in the *Journal of Gerontology* comparing an Eden Alternative home after one year with a traditional nursing home found no measurable improvement in residents or in cost of care after one year. In fact, the Eden site actually had worse outcomes as far as the number of falls and of residents with nutritional problems. "However, qualitative observations at the Eden site indicated that the change was positive for many staff as well as residents, suggesting that it may take longer than a year to demonstrate improvements," the researchers concluded.[8]

Significantly, in 2005, leading researchers held an invitation-only meeting, "Pragmatic Innovations in Long-term Care," that identified areas of research that would "help inform and guide the process of change." Led by University of North Carolina researchers Philip Sloane, MD, and Sheryl Zimmerman, the gathering came up with a comprehensive research agenda. The final report concluded: "The long-term care industry is in the midst of rapid, sweeping changes, which are anticipated to increase in momentum and scope over the coming decade; . . . given the strength of current grassroots movements for change, the time is ripe for new research." As the culture-change movement grows, we can thus expect growing interest from the research community.

"It can't last."

In 2005, a shudder went through the universe of culture-change advocates. Crestview, long considered a leading light in "person-centered care" had lost its Medicaid and Medicare certification for having so many deficiencies that surveyors no longer considered it a safe place for people to live. The drastic decline in quality occurred within a year after Eric and Margie Haider left Crestview for Florida to continue their work in transformative long-term care. According to news accounts, Crestview underwent a rapid succession of administrators, and many staff members lost their jobs. Crestview nearly was forced to close, but at this writing Medicaid certification had since been reinstated, and it has survived.

At nearly the same time the Crestview drama was unfolding, another early pioneering home, Evergreen in Oshkosh, was also dealing with the loss of its longtime administrator, David Green. After twenty-nine years leading the transformation of Evergreen, David Green retired in July 2005. He and the board had methodically planned ahead for a smooth transition. "Our board guided me through a five-year succession process," he said. "The public often looks for a heroic CEO. That's foolishness. Only when you create the team can you have sustainability."

From the housekeepers to members of the board, Evergreen worked for a decade to create a sustainable culture that was resident centered, staffed by self-directed work teams. David's successor, hired from within, was already imbued with the transformative culture.

"Change starts at the top, but it can't be built on one person," said Charlene Boyd. "When we want to change behavior and culture, we have to change systemically to make them stick."

Leaders such as Charlene, David Green, and Steve Shields embrace the "servant leader" model that flips organizational hierarchy on its head. "The longer I was CEO, the less in control I was," said David Green. "It was the people on the front line making the decisions—but they have to be prepared to do it."

Steve Shields agreed. "Change has to be deep within the organization, so that everyone owns it and is proficient. The measure of a leader is how it runs when they're gone, not when they're there."

To continually deepen understanding and ownership by the staff, homes use learning circles, send staff to culture-change conferences, and continually train staff to improve their skills. Wesley Village initiated a two-day retreat for staff in a lovely rural setting for spiritual and emotional growth. The retreats are held periodically for small groups of staff across departments, and over time, every employee attends. "It's all experiential exercises," said administrator Heidi Gil. "Staff leave with more self-awareness and confidence about their inner strengths. Many tell us their lives have changed as a result. The retreats have been the most rewarding piece of the transformation." Among the comments of staff members on evaluation forms: "Love, touch, understand, and communicate are just as important to residents as physical care"; "It was truly an enlightening experience"; and "It helped me discover parts of myself that I can work on improving or changing so I can be happier and more productive at work and at home."

Administrators on the front end of change seem energized by what they are creating. They come across as problem solvers, or more accurately, they seem to enjoy being part of an organization of problem solvers.

In her thoughtful article on nursing home culture, researcher Marian Deutschman writes: "Neither a sense of pride nor competition seems to be enough of a motivator to encourage quality and excellence. For most facilities a culture change must precede this transformation to excellence because it requires an organization with innovative leadership, considerable sharing of information, building a team, soliciting suggestions from them, being politically sensitive, and sharing rewards and recognition willingly."[9]

The role of the administrator in this process cannot be overstated. Without committed leadership at the top, a culture cannot be transformed. Without a commitment to the long haul, it will not be sustained.

How then does the field of long-term care go about attracting and nurturing the extraordinary leaders required? Will fundamental change occur only in the small number of homes lucky enough to have a visionary at the top?

Such questions lead to how administrators are trained and recruited. Here, too, are promising developments. Bonnie Kantor, in her role as director of geriatrics and gerontology at Ohio State, weaves culture change and the Pioneer Network philosophy into courses for both nursing home administration and medical students. She also incorporates the concepts of culture change in a graduate-level certificate course on aging studies, taught online to students across the country. Steve Shields and a colleague teach a similar course at Kansas State University. Other educational efforts are beginning around the country.

In 2004, the American College of Health Care Administrators created "Principles of Excellence for Leaders in Long-Term Care Administration," a document that, if implemented by every administrator, would certainly make a difference. It calls on administrators to create a "culture of quality" in terms of resident life and care and working conditions. A good administrator, it noted, "creates 'home' for each resident," "emphasizes the primacy of person-centered care," and "affirms the primacy of each resident's quality of life . . . by supporting their personal growth and by promoting their intellectual and spiritual health and social well-being."[10]

Fundamental change does not happen overnight. But these are hopeful signs that it will happen over time.

Pam Elrod of Genesis describes culture change as a marathon. "You have to keep reaching back and help the people who are behind catch up a little," she said. "You want your leadership—not always the formal leadership, your informal leaders who really own it—to reach back and bring their peers forward. People think that with culture change there is some magic place that you arrive. But it looks different every place that has embarked on this journey. I hope some day people will look at a nursing home as a wonderful place to be, as opposed to a terrible place to be. We're not going away. So why not transform it?"

Chapter 13

Baby Boomers' Legacy?
Building a Movement

> The biggest force for change would be the market. If
> consumers really get on to what the difference is in these
> places, they won't want to go to the old unchanged places.
> Every blow for creating a demand for change is all to the
> good.
> —Carter Catlett Williams, nursing home reform leader

> Together we can create a culture in which it's easier to do the
> right thing.
> —Mary Pipher, *Another Country*

Cultural transformation is an idea whose time has come. What began as a dream of a handful of radical reformers is rapidly gaining acceptance as the way life should be for people in nursing homes. This is especially remarkable given how truly radical that vision is.

In his best-selling book *The Tipping Point*, Malcolm Gladwell compares the spread of social phenomena to that of an epidemic: "What must underlie successful epidemics, in the end, is a bedrock belief that change is possible, that people can radically transform their behavior or beliefs in the face of the right kind of impetus."

Within the field of long-term care, many have worked hard to create that impetus.

Steve Shields recognized early on that transformation cannot be sustained as long as nursing homes such as Meadowlark Hills are islands in a sea of institutional mediocrity. "This thing will not survive if it doesn't become normal," he said. "That's when I started taking every speaking engagement that came my way. I knew I needed to influence regulators, our associations, providers. I told myself that I was going to just speak the truth as I experienced it, and so I did." He, Bill Thomas, and other leaders dedicate more and more time to going on the road, preaching the gospel of transformative change.

I called Richard Peck, long-time editor of *Nursing Homes* magazine, to see if their voices were being heard. Peck's magazine goes to fifty thousand long-term care managers and directors of nursing. "Culture change is a hot topic—not an easy topic," he said, especially for administrators who must lead the change.

He shared an anecdote he thought was revealing. He had recently attended a culture-change seminar in Ohio. A week before the event, only twenty people had signed up. But the day of the event, more than three hundred people descended from around the state. Although many expressed disbelief that such change could really happen, Peck said he sensed an openness unlike anything he'd witnessed in his fifteen years of covering the field. "In the past, they have been in a very reactive and defensive mode," he said. "Now, people are stepping up, just stepping up and doing it the way it's supposed to be done. It's a different philosophic mindset. This is new."

There are no hard numbers, yet only a fraction of the nation's nursing homes have committed themselves to fundamentally change. But the two main trade associations—the American Health Care Association/National Assisted Living Center (AHCA), representing primarily for-profits, and the American Association of Homes and Services for the Aging, representing not-for-profits, both enthusiastically endorse the tenets of culture change.

"We definitely support systemic change, and we do not support it just being a marketing effort," said Sandy Fitzler, AHCA senior director of clinical services. AHCA's *Provider* magazine regularly runs features on transformative homes, encouraging members to follow their lead. At AHCA's annual conventions, culture change is now a regular workshop topic, and in 2006, two of its four preconvention sessions were devoted to culture change.

Although many reform advocates and nonprofit leaders are skeptical that for-profit nursing homes, especially corporate-owned chains, will have the long-term commitment needed to transform, others say that the business case may be strong enough to prompt action.

Golden Gate National Senior Care (formerly Beverly Enterprises), one of the nation's largest corporate chains, is piloting small culture-change pilot projects at 23 of its 342 nursing homes. But as the new name implies, corporations are bought and sold, and such projects can lose the support of new owners. "We went through a change of ownership this year," said Patrice Acosta, senior vice president for quality of life programs. "There is a learning curve for our new executives to learn what this whole resident-centered approach is about and what does culture change mean to the organization." So far, she said, "their response has been very favorable."

As discussed earlier, Genesis HealthCare, also among the largest chains, is piloting culture change in its northeast region.

In 2005, John Erickson, founder and CEO of Erickson Communities, a rapidly growing chain of continuing-care retirement communities, hired Judah Ronch, a leading expert in culture change, to transform the assisted living and nursing homes at all Erickson communities. "In the past we were not as aggressive there as we should have been," Erickson said. "We went with more traditional. We're going to go more toward these family models, [such as] the Green Houses. You're going to see a lot of change in the nursing side, particularly in the dementia care."

Oatfield Estates is another family-owned for-profit that initiated resident-directed care on its own. Like Erickson, it hopes to spread its model nationally.

On the nonprofit side, in 2005, AAHSA and the Pioneer Network formed a "strategic alliance" to move culture change forward. "It's certainly a quickly growing trend," said Doug Pace, AAHSA's vice president for culture change, a newly created position. "What we're finding in our meetings, if you do a culture-change session, they pack the room."

Wesley Village is spreading its Planetree-based approach to others. In 2006, it held an international long-term care summit for twenty-three leaders of eleven long-term care organizations, devoted to developing the best practices for holistic, relationship-centered care and living environments.

Within the Veterans Administration, Christa Hojlo and her colleagues held a groundbreaking culture-transformation summit in 2005 that included housekeepers, aides, chaplains, dieticians, nurses, and elders from around the nation. A steering committee has been formed to weave a new culture into VA nursing homes, as part of every region's strategic planning process. Christa explains why they prefer the term "cultural transformation" to "culture change." "Change can be superficial—change can be a change in policy, in dress, in procedures," she says. "Change isn't necessarily a paradigm shift. What we're talking about is a paradigm shift. It's transformative. You don't do business as you did before. Here, we're talking about a fundamental transformation, at the heart level."

Culture-change leaders have paved the way for others to move forward. In 2006, Steve Shields and LaVrene Norton completed "Household Matters," a tool kit that includes a book, *In Pursuit of the Sunbeam,* a complete guide to creating and sustaining change.

The web-based My Innerview (*myinnerview.com*) offers long-term care leaders practical advice on culture change and on improving quality of life and care for residents.

Foundations such as the Retirement Research Foundation, Commonwealth Fund, and Robert Wood Johnson are supporting research and pilot projects to encourage culture change to spread. Robert Wood Johnson in 2005 awarded $10 million to support a Green House initiative across the country.

The federal bureaucracy has also given culture change its blessing. Surveyors are told to accept innovation, rather than penalize it, if residents' quality of life is enhanced. At the same time, Quality Improvement Organizations work with nursing homes in each state to create exemplary models that others can emulate.

State long-term care ombudsmen, who respond to complaints by residents and families and who advocate on their behalf, now see cultural transformation as a way to overcome decades of abuse and neglect. "I started promoting this movement through local trainings and establishing regional coalitions," said Neyna Johnson, deputy state long-term care ombudsman for Illinois and Pioneer Network board member. "We now have a statewide coalition to continue to educate and empower families and residents on different practices and approaches of culture change."

In Virginia, the ombudsman office also launched a statewide Culture Change Coalition, one of many such coalitions around the nation. "We decided that part of our mission was to spread awareness to begin to light the flame of culture change," said Joani Latimer, state ombudsman.

In Maryland, family caregivers organized Voices for Quality Care. "We feel culture change is the only thing we see on the horizon that will improve things," said coalition chair Kate Ricks. "We see a real need to give family councils and residents a place at the table and make them equal partners." In 2006, Voices for Quality Care organized seven culture-change conferences around the state for family members, staff, and regulators.

The bipartisan National Commission on Quality Long-Term Care was also established in 2005 to work toward a "bold vision" for the future and tackle such issues as public financing, workforce development, personal dignity, healthy aging, and the role of technology. Making fundamental change in such a complex system is hard work, said Vincent Mor, a long-time gerontology researcher at Brown University, who directs the commission.

> Because it's hard, most people don't want to think about it. It's too easy for us as a society to blame the bad nursing home operator. We have to blame ourselves. It's a matter of investment—not necessarily more cash, but more personal effort. I actually think that Americans are ready for

some significant social leadership, and we're just not getting it. Somebody has to say, "Listen, this is important." The baby boomers owe the country some kind of long-term care policy, just like the Depression gave us Social Security, and the Greatest Generation gave us Medicare. Baby boomers need to give us a legacy, and long-term care should be what it is.

Defeating Denial

When I tell other baby boomers about the movement to transform eldercare, they invariably respond, "Quick—change it before I get there!" While I appreciate the sentiment, the assumption that someone else will make the change, as Mor suggests, is misplaced. Only a concerted push by society will undo half a century of institutional culture. The public must demand it—not only those whose loved ones move to a nursing home, but also elders themselves in retirement communities and in advocacy groups; citizens, by becoming active in statewide culture-change coalitions; volunteers, by breaking down the barriers and forming real relationships with elders.

The hospice movement demonstrates how a compelling mission can draw volunteers. Just as community volunteers aid people at the end of life, they can become involved on a much broader scale in long-term care settings. As P. K. Beville discovered with her Second Wind Dreams project, volunteers enthusiastically take responsibility for providing meaningful experiences for elders who otherwise would not have them. Members of the public can play a significant role in changing the culture of isolation that exists in so many nursing homes and assisted-living centers.

Those who seek care for their relatives and elders must themselves demand the best. "You wouldn't check into a hotel and tolerate not having the right bedding," said Elinor Ginzler, coauthor of *Caring for Your Parents: The Complete AARP Guide.* "But people assume they can't ask for quality in the nursing homes. They need to think of themselves in the same way as a customer."

Ginzler had just returned from a trip to Nebraska, where she had spoken at a ribbon cutting for a new Green House. "If we have any sense at all, this will become not the exception but the rule over time," she said. "It really is amazing."

AARP is beginning to feature stories of transformative homes in its publications, which go to thirty-five million members. One hopes the organization will use its muscle to advocate strongly on behalf of deep culture change.

"The one point that will bring this about is public pressure," said Nancy Zweibel of the Retirement Research Foundation. "If people learn to expect that they can get this kind of care for a loved one, providers will have to do this."

Perhaps the greatest barrier to change is our mass delusional denial of aging and death. As long as our society views young adulthood as the pinnacle of life stages, elders will not live in places any of us would want to be. "Until we change the culture of aging, we're going to have a hard time changing the culture of long-term care," said Bonnie Kantor of Ohio State University. "Until people understand there's always, always something you can do to make someone healthier, that decline and disability are not to be expected, until we understand that and embrace it, they're not going to be looking at long-term care as a place for development."

Although the business of "anti-aging" products still thrives, there are hints that such a cultural shift may be beginning. For example, a new internet-based advice column, Elder Wisdom Circle, links five hundred volunteers, aged 60 to 103, with younger people who want practical advice on everything from romance and children to gardening, careers, home, and in-laws. The organization's weekly advice column is featured in major media outlets, and its website receives 60,000 to 75,000 visitors a month.

Other nonprofit organizations are cropping up, dedicated to envisioning a better model of growing old. The Memorial SAGE-ing Center, at Memorial Hospital in South Bend, Indiana, offers facilitator-training workshops for professionals and lay leaders on such topics as "Facing My Mortality," "Elders as Healers," and "Images of Aging."

New book titles include *Earth's Elders: The Wisdom of the World's Oldest People, My Time: Making the Most of the Bonus Decades after 50*, and *The Mature Mind: The Positive Power of the Aging Brain*.

The video *Almost Home*, which documents the challenges faced by a Wisconsin nursing home trying to transform, was a phenomenal success. According to producer Brad Lichtenstein, one million people saw the film, which aired 887 times on two hundred public television stations. Some four thousand DVDs of the film were distributed. "We have shown the film at literally dozens of conferences, hundreds of community screenings, and a screening on Capitol Hill," Brad said. NCCNHR and AAHSA also held nationwide conference calls on culture change for people who had seen the film. Much of this wide audience was generated through the internet.

Another video, *Brave New Home: Changing the Culture of Nursing Home Care*, was produced in Washington State and aired on public television stations there.

The news media is also picking up the story, with major media, including

National Public Radio, *Newsweek,* the *New York Times*, and the *Washington Post*, among many other outlets, covering transformational homes.

W e don't know what the future holds for those of us looking ahead to old age—only that it will look different. Technology alone will allow many of us to stay in our homes longer. The "universal design" movement in architecture is creating homes that work for older people and those with disabilities. Adjustable countertops, curtain rods, light switches, and shower stalls accommodate people in wheelchairs. Long-distance caregivers sitting at their home computers can check in on a frail parent through sophisticated new monitoring systems. Engineers are even working on robotic aides that can fetch a glass of water for an older person who has difficulty getting around.

More and more people who once would have ended up in a nursing home now move to assisted living or board-and-care homes, or receive home-health services. So-called NORCs (naturally occurring retirement communities) are springing up. These are neighborhoods, small towns, even trailer parks, with a high density of older people, who find ways to have services brought to them, allowing them to stay put. Others envision creating their own Green Houses where a group of friends might share space and hire caregivers as needed.

"I don't have all the solutions to old age," said Barbara Thomas, administrator of Kendal at Oberlin. "I don't know what's going to happen with new medications coming out, new surgeries that are possible, new technologies. But I do know that with an engaged population, no matter what problems we face, we're going to face it together."

John Glaser, director of the Center for Healthcare Reform, a Catholic nonprofit organization advocating fundamental change in our nation's healthcare system, believes sweeping social change begins with an exploration of shared values. The civil rights and women's suffrage movements, he argues, did not begin with technicalities about the design of the ballot box. Regulators and policymakers did not start these movements. They instead grew out of a moral conviction that a great wrong needed to be righted. Their aims, once highly controversial and wrenching to society, are now accepted by virtually everyone as fair and just. The time is ripe for a similar national consciousness-raising regarding the lives of elders.

Karen Schoeneman, looking back only nine years to the birth of the Pioneer Network, is an optimist. "Thirty-three people decided to crack the world," she said. "We decided to change the culture, to start a new civil rights movement for people who live in nursing homes. We're baby boomers, for the most part. We remember the civil rights movement, we remember the women's rights movement. Now there's ten thousand of us. There are hundreds of leaders taking back the message. They're all welcome at the gathering place. It's a beautiful thing to see."

Regardless of how we envision meeting our needs as we grow old, the lessons of these pioneers will hold true. Elders' needs are our own: to live in dignity, in an environment of home, in a community of nurture and love, leading a life that has meaning.

In a rousing speech at the 2004 Pioneer Network national conference, titled "There's No Place Like Home," Bill Thomas said:

> What kind of society builds seventeen thousand nursing homes? It's the kind of society that's lost its mooring.
>
> We have to get good at talking about the nursing home. The nursing home is where we practice the art of knowing, the place where we nurture hope, where you build a beacon of light where you never expected to find a beacon of light.
>
> But we're after something bigger—the right and opportunity to have a life worth living that extends into the last years, days, and minutes of life. We are the people who stand up for the frailest, sickest, most forgetful people in our society. The system we're about changing is American culture.

Epilogue

I sit in the living room of a Green House in Tupelo and absorb life here. If going to a nursing home meant this, would people live in fear and dread? I would not. People were sick and had trouble moving, and some were more than a century old. Many were clearly living in a different sort of reality. But the house was full of life, of warmth, of love. I saw nothing to fear.

A food-service worker from the campus enters and comes immediately to hug Mrs. Dunn, who is chatting with me. Mrs. Dunn tells me she was raised on a farm outside Tupelo. She spent her working life in factories and babysitting.

"I make something called a sad cake out of Bisquick—I want to make it for an upcoming family reunion," she says. The shahbazim would make sure she has the ingredients and give her any assistance she might need to bake it.

On one wall are photos of the original residents of this Green House, including one of a young Mrs. Dunn. Today, she wears a bright red top and blue jeans. She is going to the mall with Ida Cummings, a lovely young shahbaz, and two other elders.

Ida leans over and kisses "Mrs. Thomas," an elder who seems one of the most debilitated. Mrs. Dunn tells me softly that she hopes she never gets like Mrs. Thomas, who apparently is unable to hear or to speak and who has little use of her limbs.

Betty Mae Pryor, a nurse, goes from room to room, doling out medications. She has red hair and is always joking or singing. She is dressed in jeans and a t-shirt with a Christian theme. She has a pleasing voice, like the solo in a church choir. She sings "We Will Follow the Steps of Jesus" as she makes her rounds. She knocks on a bedroom door, and a man's voice greets her. "Good morning, honey. You look nice today."

Betty Mae tells him he should go to the mall with the others. "You might see some good-looking women," she says.

"He can see them right here," Mrs. Dunn chimes in.

Betty Mae helps the shahbazim by lugging in snacks and a box of orange juice to the kitchen from the front porch. She stops and tells Mrs. Dunn with mock sternness, "If you're not careful I'm going to give you sugar on the cheek" (Mississippi-speak for a kiss).

"I *like* sugar on the cheek," Mrs. Dunn declares.

Ida wheels out Sara Biddle, who sits next to me at the table. Ida helps her eat a bowl of Wheat Chex. Sara Biddle's room has pretty matching yellow-flowered sheets and curtains. There are many crosses and family photos on the walls.

Later I return to the house to say good-bye. Mrs. Thomas's daughter calls, and Ida tells her about the trip to the mall. She tells her what Mrs. Thomas wore. "She didn't go to sleep once," she says into the phone. "I think it was a real good idea to take her out." Mrs. Thomas ate a big lunch and was alert and looking at everyone, she says.

The other resident who went to the mall, "Vivian," had once been a champion fiddle player in Alabama, I am told. I asked her how the mall was. She laughs and says, "It's there—same as always."

Mrs. Dunn is pleased with her purchase—a silk pillowcase.

Another shahbaz, Dale Letson, had been a tool-and-die maker but was laid off when the company closed down. "When this opportunity came open, I changed fields. I love it. I think I've been looking for this all my life," she says. At sixty-three, she is one of the older shahbazim. She hopes to go to nursing school. "If I didn't have responsibilities at home, I'd be here as much as they'd let me," she says. "Most of all, I love the elders and making them as comfortable as possible. I love to cook, and making sure they have the things they need."

Ida's daughter drops by after school. She runs over to Mrs. Dunn, and they hug. Mrs. Dunn and Ida tell me they like to go to yard sales together.

It's time for me to leave. Dale hugs me. Mrs. Dunn hugs me. Then they hug each other.

"We believe in hugs, don't we," Mrs. Dunn says, smiling. She hugs me tightly once more and tells me softly, "God bless you."

Appendixes

A. Resident's Rights Granted by the Nursing Home Reform Act

The Right to Be Fully Informed, including:

The right to be informed of all services available as well as the charge for each service;

The right to have a copy of the nursing home's rules and regulations, including a written copy of their rights;

The right to be informed of the address and telephone number of the State Ombudsman, State licensure office, and other advocacy groups;

The right to see the State survey reports of the nursing home and the home's plan of correction;

The right to be notified in advance of any plans to change their room or roommate;

The right to daily communication in their language;

The right to assistance if they have a sensory impairment.

The Right to Participate in Their Own Care, including:

The right to receive adequate or appropriate care;

The right to be informed of any changes in their medical condition;

The right to participate in planning their treatment, care, and discharge;

The right to refuse medication and treatment;

The right to refuse chemical and physical restraints;

The right to review their medical record.

The Right to Make Independent Choices, including:

The right to make independent personal decisions, such as what to wear and
  how to spend free time;
The right to reasonable accommodation of their needs and preferences by the
  nursing home;
The right to choose their own physician;
The right to participate in community activities, both inside and outside the
  nursing home;
The right to organize and participate in a Resident Council.

The Right to Privacy and Confidentiality, including:

The right to private and unrestricted communication with any person of their
  choice;
The right to privacy in treatment and in the care of their personal needs;
The right to confidentiality regarding their medical, personal, or financial
  affairs.

The Right to Dignity, Respect, and Freedom, including:

The right to be treated with the fullest measure of consideration, respect, and
  dignity;
The right to be free from mental and physical abuse, corporal punishment,
  involuntary seclusion, and physical and chemical restraints;
The right to self-determination.

The Right to Security of Possessions, including:

The right to manage their own financial affairs;
The right to file a complaint with the State survey and certification agency for
  abuse, neglect, or misappropriation of their property if the nursing home
  is handling their financial affairs;
The right to be free from charge for services covered by Medicaid or
  Medicare.

Rights during Transfers and Discharges, including:

The right to remain in the nursing facility unless a transfer or discharge: is necessary to meet the resident's welfare; is appropriate because the resident's health has improved and the resident no longer requires nursing home care; is needed to protect the health and safety of other residents or staff; is required because the resident has failed, after reasonable notice, to pay the facility charge for an item or service provided at the resident's request;

The right to receive notice of transfer or discharge. A thirty-day notice is required. The notice must include the reason for transfer or discharge, the effective date, the location to which the resident is transferred or discharged, a statement of the right to appeal, and the name, address, and telephone number of the state long-term care ombudsman;

The right to a safe transfer or discharge through sufficient preparation by the nursing home.

The Right to Complain, including:

The right to present grievances to the staff of the nursing home, or to any other person, without fear of reprisal;

The right to prompt efforts by the nursing home to resolve grievances.

The Right to Visits, including:

The right to immediate access by a resident's personal physician and representatives from the health department and ombudsman programs;

The right to immediate access by their relatives and for others subject to reasonable restriction with the resident's permission;

The right to reasonable visits by organizations or individuals providing health, social, legal, or other services.

B. Pioneer Network Values and Principles

Know each person

Each person can and does make a difference

Relationship is the fundamental building block of a transformed culture

Respond to spirit, as well as mind and body

Risk taking is a normal part of life

Put person before task

All elders are entitled to self-determination wherever they live

Community is the antidote to institutionalization

Do unto others as you would have them do unto you—yes, the Golden Rule

Promote the growth and development of all

Shape and use the potential of the environment in all its aspects: physical, organizational, psycho/social/spiritual

Practice self-examination, searching for new creativity and opportunities for doing better

Recognize that culture change and transformation are not destinations but a journey, always a work in progress

C. The Eden Alternative Principles

1. The three plagues of loneliness, helplessness and boredom account for the bulk of suffering among our Elders.
2. An Elder-centered community commits to creating a Human Habitat where life revolves around close and continuing contact with plants, animals and children. It is these relationships that provide the young and old alike with a pathway to a life worth living.
3. Loving companionship is the antidote to loneliness. Elders deserve easy access to human and animal companionship.
4. An Elder-centered community creates opportunity to give as well as receive care. This is the antidote to helplessness.
5. An Elder-centered community imbues daily life with variety and spontaneity by creating an environment in which unexpected and unpredictable interactions and happenings can take place. This is the antidote to boredom.
6. Meaningless activity corrodes the human spirit. The opportunity to do things that we find meaningful is essential to human health.
7. Medical treatment should be the servant of genuine human caring, never its master.
8. An Elder-centered community honors its Elders by de-emphasizing top-down bureaucratic authority, seeking instead to place the maximum possible decision-making authority into the hands of the Elders or into the hands of those closest to them.
9. Creating an Elder-centered community is a never-ending process. Human growth must never be separated from human life.
10. Wise leadership is the lifeblood of any struggle against the three plagues. For it, there can be no substitute.

D. Planetree Continuing Care: Creating Relationship-Centered Caring Environments

Human Interactions

Planetree is about human beings caring for one another. A Planetree continuing care community fosters caring relationships among residents, families, employees, and volunteers by emphasizing self-awareness and personal accountability. Staff retreats provide an understanding of the needs of older adults and sensitize staff to life from the resident's perspective, while building team relationship skills through experiential exercises. Ongoing seminars for residents and staff offer tools for communicating positively, maintaining authentic relationships, and managing conflicts in a dignified manner.

Enhancement of Life's Journey

A Planetree continuing care community offers opportunities for personal growth, self-expression, and the fulfillment of individual dreams. Planetree supports individuals who provide volunteer service to the communities where they live and work. Through group discussions, journal writing and a life stories program, individuals have opportunities to review their life, clarify what they value, and determine personal goals. In a life stories program, a trained volunteer interviews a resident and writes a short story that captures some of the pivotal events in that resident's life. These short stories are shared with caregivers, enabling them to see each resident as a whole person rather than primarily as "someone needing services," and creating bonds between individuals that deepen mutual respect, trust, and concern.

Independence, Dignity, and Choice

A Planetree continuing care community offers a range of options that support an individual's autonomy, lifestyle, and interests. Residents are encouraged to remain as independent as possible. When planning services, staff members interview the resident and/or the responsible family member to discuss expectations and preferences so that services can be personalized. A residents' association provides a channel for communication and input. Staff training emphasizes respect for privacy and personal space.

Family, Friends, and Social Support Networks

Social support and loving relationships are vital to good health. A Planetree continuing care community surrounds residents with people whom they can depend on and encourages individuals to actively build trusting relationships.

It enables residents to maintain their connections to family and friends by providing unrestricted visiting hours, flexible schedules, and convenient access to telephone and e-mail. There is a process to match residents with their neighbors, and staff with their peers, especially during times of need. Support groups help individuals cope with transitions, illness, loss, grief, and stress. A care partner program actively involves family members and friends in planning and providing care.

Spirituality

Planetree recognizes that spirituality is essential to a fulfilling life. A Planetree community provides opportunities to strengthen the relationship with one's faith and inner resources. Residents and staff have opportunities for worship, prayer, meditation, and ceremonies such as an annual Blessing of the Hands that celebrates the caring spirit of the staff. In addition, there are educational programs about spirituality and opportunities to discuss, both privately with clergy and in groups, the meaning and spiritual dimensions of life and one's personal beliefs and values. Pastoral care is available for residents and staff for routine needs as well as for times of stress such as illness or the death of a loved one.

Paths to Well-Being

A Planetree continuing care community provides innovative programs for residents and staff that maintain health and fitness and that complement western scientific medical care. Wellness programs include prevention and management of chronic diseases and convenient access to vision, hearing, dental, and other specialized services. There are exercise facilities with equipment designed for seniors and personalized programs for strength, balance and fitness training based on individual assessments and benchmarks. Naturopathic medicine, aromatherapy, guided imagery, massage, yoga, and meditation classes are offered.

Empowerment through Information and Education

A Planetree continuing care community gives residents and staff the information necessary to understand their situation and maximize their physical, psychological, and financial well-being. There are educational programs about preventing and coping with diseases, a resource library, and computers with internet access. A Continuous Quality Improvement process throughout the organization encourages staff at all levels, residents, and family members to work together to solve problems and exceed quality standards. Staff are trained to take the initiative in resolving issues that arise with resident services.

Nutritional and Nurturing Aspects of Food

Planetree recognizes that eating is not only essential to physical health, but is also a source of pleasure, comfort, and fellowship. A Planetree dining program enhances the social aspects of meals while serving delicious fresh food that is attractively presented in a pleasant environment. A full-service dining program offers changing, nutritionally-balanced menus with choices of entrees and side dishes, including heart-healthy choices, that are responsive to individual preferences. Mealtimes are flexible and healthy snacks are available at all times. The dining program includes special events, holiday meals, parties, and picnics for residents and staff.

Activities and Entertainment

Planetree recognizes that people need opportunities for camaraderie, laughter, and creativity. A Planetree continuing care community offers a variety of activities that include classes, discussions, concerts, parties, outings, intergenerational programs, and family events. To broaden the relationships between staff and residents, staff participate in special resident activities. Transportation accommodates residents who wish to attend off-site events and to volunteer for local organizations. For animal lovers, pets visit regularly. An employee committee plans activities that enliven the workplace and encourage fellowship.

Environment Conducive to Quality Living

Planetree recognizes that the physical environment has a tremendous effect on the well-being of residents and staff: The design of a Planetree continuing care community incorporates public and private space, residential décor, natural light, and views of nature. An uncluttered environment facilitates movement and communication, creating a feeling of "safe shelter." There is a library, and space for group activities, social gatherings, and worship. Common areas feature artwork, music, plants, and fish tanks. Flower gardens, fountains, labyrinths, and outdoor sitting areas allow individuals to experience the relaxing, invigorating, and meditative aspects of nature. The design and operations provide for the safety and security of residents, staff, and visitors while enhancing the quality of life.

Notes

INTRODUCTION

1. Benyamin Schwarz, *Nursing Home Design: Consequences of Employing the Medical Model* (New York: Garland, 1996), 37.

CHAPTER 1

1. Rosalie A. Kane, "Long-Term Care and a Good Quality of Life: Bringing Them Closer Together," *The Gerontologist* 41, no. 3 (2001): 295.
2. Bill Thomas pointed out this comparison to me. The number of nursing homes came from the Administration on Aging, *www.aoa.gov/prof/notes/notes_nursing_homes_pf.asp*. On McDonald's numbers, e-mail communication from McDonald's USA, March 21, 2006.
3. For nursing home employee figures, see *www.ahca.org*. According to Wal-Mart's website, *www.walmartfacts.com,* there were 1.3 million Wal-Mart employees in the United States as of February 2007. For the cost of nursing homes: Ellen O'Brien, "Medicaid's Coverage of Nursing Home Costs: Asset Shelter for the Wealthy or Essential Safety Net?" Issue Brief, Georgetown University Long-Term Care Financing Project, May 2005. For elder population figures: U.S. Census Bureau, "65+ in the United States: 2005," December 2005. For projected number of nursing home residents: National Center for Health Statistics, "The Changing Profile of Nursing Home Residents: 1985–1997," March 2001.
4. Vincent Mor, Jacqueline Zinn, Joseph Angelelli, Joan M. Teno, and Susan C. Miller, "Driven to Tiers: Socioeconomic and Racial Disparities in the Quality of Nursing Home Care," *Milbank Quarterly* 82, no. 2 (2004): 227–56. On resident costs: Genworth Financial 2006 Cost of Care Survey, March 2006, at *longtermcare.genworth.com/overview/what_is_ltc.jsp*. For numbers of for-profit homes, see *www.ahca.org*.
5. U.S. Government Accountability Office, "Nursing Homes: Despite Increased Oversight, Challenges Remain in Ensuring High-Quality Care and Resident Safety," GAO-06-117, December 2005, 4.

6. Bruce C. Vladeck, *Unloving Care: The Nursing Home Tragedy* (New York: Basic Books, 1980), 4.

7. Bruce C. Vladeck, "*Unloving Care* Revisited: The Persistence of Culture," in *Culture Change in Long-Term Care*, ed. Audrey S. Weiner and Judah L. Ronch (Binghamton, N.Y.: Haworth Press, 2003), 3.

8. Pew Research Center, "Baby Boomers: From the Age of Aquarius to the Age of Responsibility," Dec. 8, 2005, *pewresearch.org/social/pack.php?PackID=6*.

9. Herbert Shore, "New Ideas in Institutional Care," *Professional Nursing Home*, June 1966, 40.

10. Karen Stevenson, *www.elderweb.com*. Other sources on which I drew for the history of nursing homes include Schwarz, *Nursing Home Design*; Vladeck, *Unloving Care*; Colleen L. Johnson and Leslie A. Grant, *The Nursing Home in American Society* (Baltimore: Johns Hopkins University Press, 1985); Charles W. Lidz, Lynn Fischer, and Robert M. Arnold, *The Erosion of Autonomy in Long-Term Care* (New York: Oxford University Press, 1992).

11. Vladeck, *Unloving Care*, 31.

12. See *www.nccnhr.org* for a history of the organization.

13. For the 1989 figure, Diana Johnson, "Restraint-Free Care: A Look Back," *Nursing Homes*, September 1995; for the 2006 figure, *www.medicare. gov/NHCompare*.

14. Vladeck, "*Unloving Care* Revisited," 6.

15. GE Center for Financial Learning, survey on myths and misperceptions about long-term care, released September 25, 2002. MetLife Mature Market Institute poll, July 14, 2004. For the 50–70 percent: MetLife Mature Market Institute, "The Media Reality Check: Content Analysis of Recent News Coverage of Long-Term Care Insurance," October 2004, estimated at least 50 percent; the GE poll estimated 70 percent.

16. Kaiser HealthPoll Report, May–June 2005, *www.kff.org/healthreport*.

17. Joyce Horner, *That Time of Year: A Chronicle of Life in a Nursing Home* (University of Massachusetts Press, 1982), 185.

18. Department of Health and Human Services, Office of Inspector General, "State Ombudsman Data: Nursing Home Complaints," July 2003, *www.oig. hhs.gov*.

19. Robert L. Rubinstein and Patricia A. Parmelee, "Attachment to Place and the Representation of the Life Course by the Elderly," in *Place Attachment*, ed. Irwin Altman and Setha M. Low (New York: Plenum Press, 1992), 147.

20. "Dear Abby," *Washington Post*, April 1, 2003, and responses April 11.

21. Floyd Skloot, *In the Shadow of Memory* (Lincoln: University of Nebraska Press, 2003), 51.

22. From Beth Baker, "Old Age in Brave New Settings," *Washington Post*, Health section, July 16, 2002.

CHAPTER 2

1. Rubinstein and Parmelee, "Attachment to Place," 155.

2. Loren Eiseley, "The Brown Wasps," *The Night Country* (New York: Scribner's, 1971), 229.

3. Erving Goffman, *Asylums* (Garden City, N.Y.: Anchor Books, 1961), 6.
4. Witold Rybczynski, *Home: A Short History of an Idea* (New York: Penguin Books, 1986), 20–21.
5. Thomas Edward Gass, *Nobody's Home: Candid Reflections of a Nursing Home Aide* (Ithaca, N.Y.: Cornell University Press, 2004), 54.
6. Ibid., 78.
7. Johnson and Grant, *The Nursing Home in American Society*, 77–78.
8. Mindy Thompson Fullilove, "Psychiatric Implications of Displacement: Contributions from the Psychology of Place," *American Journal of Psychiatry* 153, no. 12 (1996): 1518.
9. Johnson and Grant, *The Nursing Home in American Society*, 69.
10. Judith T. Carboni, "Homelessness among the Institutionalized Elderly," *Journal of Gerontological Nursing* 16, no. 7 (1990): 34.
11. Tom Kitwood, *Dementia Reconsidered: The Person Comes First* (Buckingham, UK: Open University Press, 1997), 134.
12. John E. Morley and Joseph H. Flaherty, "Putting the 'Home' Back in Nursing Home," *Journal of Gerontology Series A*, 57A, no. 7 (2002): M419.
13. Rubinstein and Parmelee, "Attachment to Place," 143.

CHAPTER 3

1. Gass, *Nobody's Home*, 34.
2. Carrie Knowles, *The Last Childhood: A Family Story of Alzheimer's* (New York: Three Rivers Press, 2000), 152.
3. Candice Choi, "Seniors Moving Out of Nursing Home System," Associated Press, June 14, 2006.
4. Johnson and Grant, *The Nursing Home in American Society*, 74.
5. Ibid.
6. Barbara J. Patterson, "The Process of Social Support: Adjusting to Life in a Nursing Home," *Journal of Advanced Nursing* 21, no. 4 (1995): 683.
7. Rosalie A. Kane, "Personal Autonomy for Residents in Long-Term Care: Concepts and Issues of Measurement," in *The Concept and Measurement of Quality of Life in the Frail Elderly*, ed. James Birren et al. (Burlington, Mass.: Academic Press, 1991), 328.
8. Robert M. Sapolsky, *Why Zebras Don't Get Ulcers* (New York: Henry Holt, 2004), 397.
9. Gass, *Nobody's Home*, 151.
10. See *www.fda.gov/cdrh/beds*.
11. Karen Hellwig, "Alternatives to Restraints: What Patients and Caregivers Should Know," *Home Healthcare Nurse* 18, no. 6 (2000): 402.
12. See *www.medicare.gov/NHCompare*.
13. Marilyn J. Rantz and Marcia K. Flesner, *Person-Centered Care: A Model for Nursing Homes* (Washington, D.C.: American Nurses Association, 2004), 24–25.
14. Connie Vaughn Roush and Josephine E. Cox, "The Meaning of Home: How it Shapes the Practice of Home and Hospice Care," *Home Healthcare Nurse* 18, no. 6 (2000): 393.

CHAPTER 4

1. American Health Care Association, "Results of the 2002 AHCA Survey of Nursing Staff Vacancy and Turnover in Nursing Homes," February 12, 2003; Department of Health and Human Services, Office of Inspector General, "State Ombudsman Data: Nursing Home Complaints," July 2003, *www.oig. hhs.gov*

2. For general statistics and income level, National Clearinghouse on the Direct Care Workforce, "Who Are Direct-Care Workers?" Fact Sheet, September 2004, *www.directcareclearinghouse.org*; for median hourly earnings, U.S. Bureau of Labor Statistics, "Occupational Outlook Handbook, 2006–2007," *www. bls.gov/oco/print/ocos165.*

3. Donald L. Redfoot, "'We Shall Travel On': Quality of Care, Economic Development, and the International Migration of Long-Term Care Workers," AARP Public Policy Institute, October 2005, *www.aarp. org/research/longtermcare/quality/.*

4. Gass, *Nobody's Home*, 74–75.

5. Institute for the Future of Aging Services, "Keeping Frontline Workers in Long-Term Care: Research Results of an Intervention," December 2003, *www.futureofaging.org.*

6. Lori L. Jervis, "The Pollution of Incontinence and the Dirty Work of Caregiving in a U.S. Nursing Home," *Medical Anthropology Quarterly* 15, no. 1 (2001): 84.

7. For the administrator survey, Wonita Janzen, "Long-Term Care for Older Adults: The Role of the Family," *Journal of Gerontological Nursing* 27, no. 2 (2001): 41. The U.S. Bureau of Labor Statistics finding and the violence-prevention study are cited by Donna M. Gates, Evelyn Fitzwater, and Ursula Meyer, "Violence against Caregivers in Nursing Homes: Expected, Tolerated, and Accepted," *Journal of Gerontological Nursing* 25, no. 4 (1999): 12.

8. Service Employees International Union, "Caring till It Hurts: How Nursing Home Work Is Becoming the Most Dangerous Job in America," 2d ed., 1997, at *www.seiu.org/docUploads/caring_till_it_hurts.pdf.*

9. Timothy Diamond, *Making Gray Gold: Narratives of Nursing Home Care* (Chicago: University of Chicago Press, 1982), 175.

10. Ibid.

11. Ibid., 173.

12. Nursing Home Community Coalition of New York State, "What Makes for a Good Working Condition for Nursing Home Staff: What Do Direct Care Workers Have to Say?" *www.nhccnys.org*, June 2003.

13. Institute for the Future of Aging Services, "Keeping Frontline Workers in Long-Term Care."

14. Meg LaPorte, "Overworked DONs in Need of Relief," *Provider*, June 2006, 11.

15. Paraprofessional Healthcare Institute, "Direct-Care Health Workers: The Unnecessary Crisis in Long-Term Care," Domestic Strategy Group of the Aspen Institute, January 2001, *www.paraprofessional.org/Sections/resources. htm*; National Citizens' Coalition for Nursing Home Reform, "Nursing Home Staffing: A Guide for Residents, Families, Friends, and Caregivers," May 2002, cites studies related to levels of staffing and incidence of risk.

16. Institute of Medicine, *Nursing Staff in Hospitals and Nursing Homes: Is It Adequate?* (Washington, D.C.: National Academy Press, 1996).

17. Dorie Seavey, "The Cost of Frontline Turnover in Long-Term Care," Institute for the Future of Aging Services, Better Jobs Better Care Program, October 2004, at *www.bjbc.org/content/docs/TOCostReport.pdf.*

18. Nancy Foner, *The Caregiving Dilemma: Work in an American Nursing Home* (Berkeley: University of California Press, 1994), 81, 88.

19. David Farrell, Barbara Frank, Cathie Brady, Marguerite McLaughlin, and Ann Gray, "A Case for Consistent Assignment," *Provider*, June 2006, 47.

20. Barbara J. Bowers, Sarah Esmond, and Nora Jacobson, "Turnover Reinterpreted: CNAs Talk about Why They Leave," *Journal of Gerontological Nursing* 29, no. 3 (2003): 39, 40.

21. Ibid., 40.

22. Robyn I. Stone, with Joshua M. Wiener, "Who Will Care for Us? Addressing the Long-Term Care Crisis," Urban Institute and American Association of Homes and Services for the Aging, October 2001, 5, *www.rwjf.org/files/publications/other/CareForUs.pdf.*

23. Susan C. Eaton, "Beyond 'Unloving Care': Linking Human Resource Management and Patient Care Quality in Nursing Homes," *International Journal of Human Resource Management* 11, no. 3 (2000): 591–616.

24. Karen Pennington, Jill Scott, and Kathy Magilvy, "The Role of Certified Nursing Assistants in Nursing Homes," *JONA, The Journal of Nursing Administration* 33, no. 11 (2003): 583.

25. Farrell et al., "A Case for Consistent Assignment," 51.

26. Sarah Greene Burger, Jeanie Kayser-Jones, and Julie Prince Bell, "Food for Thought: Preventing/Treating Malnutrition and Dehydration," *Contemporary Longterm Care*, April 2001, 24.

27. Cathy A. Pelletier, "What Do Certified Nurse Assistants Actually Know about Dysphagia and Feeding Nursing Home Residents?" *American Journal of Speech-Language Pathology* 13 (2004): 99–104.

28. Burger, Kayser-Jones, and Bell, "Food for Thought," 26.

29. See Beth Baker, "Old Age in Brand New Settings," *Washington Post*, July 16, 2002.

30. William H. Thomas, *What Are Old People For? How Elders Will Save the World* (Acton, Mass.: VanderWyk and Burnham, 2004), 222.

31. Part of the Green House story reported in this chapter and the next first appeared in Beth Baker, "Small World," AARP Bulletin, September 2005, *www.aarp.org/bulletin/longterm/greenhouse.html.*

CHAPTER 5

The first epigraph is from Karen Bermann, "Love and Space in the Nursing Home," *Theoretical Medicine* 24 (2003): 511–23.

1. Roger S. Ulrich, "Effects of Healthcare Interior Design on Wellness: Theory and Recent Scientific Research," in *Innovations in Health Care Design*, ed. S. O. Marberry (New York: Van Nostrand Reinhold, 1995), 88–104.

2. Neva L. Crogan, "Improving Nursing Home Food Service: Uncovering the

Meaning of Food through Residents' Stories," *Journal of Gerontological Nursing* 30, no. 2 (2004): 35.

3. Northern Itasca Health Care Center, "Northern Pines Communities: A New Vision for Long Term Care," undated report.

4. Schwarz, *Nursing Home Design*, 87.

5. Carter Catlett Williams, "Days and Years in Long-Term Care: Living vs. Surviving," *Journal of Geriatric Psychiatry* 27, no. 1 (1994): 100.

CHAPTER 6

1. Craig R. Hullett, Jill J. McMillan, and Randall G. Rogan, "Caregivers' Predispositions and Perceived Organizational Expectations for the Provision of Social Support to Nursing Home Residents," *Health Communication* 12, no. 3 (2000): 278.

2. Shore, "New Ideas in Institutional Care."

3. Dominique Paulus and Beatrice Jans, "Assessing Resident Satisfaction with Institutional Living," *Journal of Gerontological Nursing* 31, no. 8 (2005): 9.

4. T. J. Hicks, Jr., "What Is Your Life Like Now? Loneliness and Elderly Individuals Residing in Nursing Homes," *Journal of Gerontological Nursing* 26, no. 8 (2000): 15–19.

5. K. B. Adams, S. Sanders, and E. Auth, "Depression and Loneliness in an Independent Living Retirement Community: Risk and Resilience Factors," *Aging and Mental Health* 8, no. 6 (2004): 475–485. Sherry M. Cummings, "Predictors of Psychological Well-Being among Assisted-Living Residents," *Health and Social Work* 27, no. 4 (2002): 293–302.

6. See Beth Baker, "RX: Friendship," *Common Boundary*, January/February 1998, 38.

7. Audrey Weiner and Sheldon L. Goldberg, "Aging in the New Millennium: What the Future Holds for Us," in *Mental Wellness in Aging: Strengths-Based Approaches,* ed. Judah L. Ronch and Joseph A. Goldfield (Baltimore: Health Professions Press, 2003), 8.

8. Study cited by Sheldon S. Tobin, "The Historical Context of 'Humanistic' Culture Change in Long-Term Care," in *Culture Change in Long-Term Care*, 62.

9. Jodi Cohn and Judith A. Sugar, "Determinants of Quality of Life in Institutions: Perceptions of Frail Older Residents, Staff, and Families," in *The Concept and Measurement of Quality of Life*, 28–49.

10. Joel Savinshinsky, "In and Out of Bounds: The Ethics of Respect in Studying Nursing Homes," in *The Culture of Long-Term Care: Nursing Home Ethnography*, ed. J. Neil Henderson and Maria D. Vesperi (Westport, Conn.: Bergin and Garvey, 1995), 96.

11. Thomas, *What Are Old People For?* 269.

12. Anthony G. Tuckett, "The Care Encounter: Pondering Caring, Honest Communication, and Control," *International Journal of Nursing Practice* 11 (2005): 77–84.

13. See, for example, Kristine Nordlie Williams, Teresa Buchhorn Ilten, and Helen Bower, "Meeting Communication Needs: Topics of Talk in the Nursing Home," *Journal of Psychosocial Nursing and Mental Health Services* 43, no. 7 (2005): 43.

14. Hicks, "What Is Your Life Like Now?" 18.

15. Catherine S. McGilton, Linda L. O'Brien-Pallas, Gerarda Darlington, Martin Evans, Francine Wynn, and Dorothy M. Pringle, "Effects of a Relationship-Enhancing Program of Care on Outcomes, *Journal of Nursing Scholarship* 35, no. 2 (2003): 155.

16. Thomas, *What Are Old People For?* 222.

CHAPTER 7

1. E-mail communication to the author from American Association of Homes and Services for the Aging, March 2006.

CHAPTER 8

1. Sharon R. Kaufman, *The Ageless Self: Sources of Meaning in Late Life* (Madison: University of Wisconsin Press, 1986), 7, 13.

2. Gene Cohen, *The Creative Age: Awakening Human Potential in the Second Half of Life* (New York: HarperCollins, 2000), 234.

3. University of Wisconsin–Eau Claire news release, November 1, 2002.

4. Clarissa A. Rentz, "Memories in the Making: Outcome-Based Evaluation of an Art Program for Individuals with Dementing Illnesses," *American Journal of Alzheimer's Disease and Other Dementias* 17, no. 3 (2002): 175–81.

5. Patterson, "The Process of Social Support," 685.

6. Robert L. Kane and Joan C. West, *It Shouldn't Be This Way: The Failure of Long-Term Care* (Nashville: Vanderbilt University Press, 2005), 107.

7. Patricia M. Burbank, "An Exploratory Study: Assessing the Meaning in Life among Older Adult Clients," *Journal of Gerontological Nursing* 18, no. 9 (1992): 19–28.

8. Kitwood, *Dementia Reconsidered*, 90.

9. Ronch and Goldfield, *Mental Wellness in Aging*, 166.

10. Patterson, "The Process of Social Support," 686.

11. Alan Dienstag, "Lessons from the Lifelines Writing Group for People in the Early Stages of Alzheimer's Disease," in *Mental Wellness in Aging*, 350.

12. Alan Beck and Aaron Katcher, *Between Pets and People: The Importance of Animal Companionship* (West Lafayette, Ind.: Purdue University Press, 1996), 150–51.

13. Harold G. Koenig, Debra K. Weiner, Bercedis L. Peterson, Keith G. Meador, and Francis J. Keefe, "Religious Coping in the Nursing Home: A Biopsychosocial Model," *International Journal of Psychiatry in Medicine* 27, no. 4 (1997): 366.

14. P. Pressman, J. S. Lyons, D. B. Larson, and J. J. Strain, "Religious Belief, Depression, and Ambulation Status in Elderly Women with Broken Hips," *American Journal of Psychiatry* 147, no. 6 (1990): 758–60.

15. Theris A. Touhy, "Nurturing Hope and Spirituality in the Nursing Home," *Holistic Nursing Practice* 15, no. 4 (2001): 48.

16. Ibid., 45.

17. Kathleen A. Bickerstaff, Carol M. Grasser, and Barbara McCabe, "How Elderly Nursing Home Residents Transcend Losses of Later Life," *Holistic Nursing Practice* 17, no. 3 (2003): 164.

18. E-mail communication with author, April 27, 2006.
19. Williams, "Days and Years in Long-Term Care," 98.

CHAPTER 9

1. Carol Levine, "The Loneliness of the Long-Term Care Giver," in *Always on Call: When Illness Turns Families into Caregivers*, ed. Carole Levine (New York: United Hospital Fund of New York, 2000), 75. Vanderbilt University Press published an expanded and updated edition of Levine's book in 2004.
2. National Alliance for Caregiving and AARP, "Caregiving in the U.S.," April 2004, *www.caregiving.org/data/04finalreport.pdf*. See also National Alliance for Family Caregiving, *www.caregiver.org*.
3. Alzheimer's Association and National Alliance for Caregiving, "Families Care: Alzheimer's Caregiving in the United States, 2004," September 2004, *www.alz. org/Resources/FactSheets/Caregiverreport.pdf*.
4. Barry J. Jacobs, "From Sadness to Pride: Seven Common Emotional Experiences of Caregiving," in *Always on Call*, 96.
5. Cynthia L. Port, Sheryl Zimmerman, Christianna S. Williams, Debra Dobbs, John S. Preisser, and Sharon Wallace Williams, "Families Filling the Gap: Comparing Family Involvement for Assisted Living and Nursing Home Residents with Dementia," *The Gerontologist* 45 supplement (2005): 87–95.
6. Ibid.
7. Cynthia L. Port, Ann L. Gruber-Baldini, Lynda Burton, Mona Baumgarten, J. Richard Hebel, Sheryl Itkin Zimmerman, and Jay Magaziner, "Resident Contact with Family and Friends Following Nursing Home Admission, *The Gerontologist* 41, no. 5 (2001): 589–96.
8. Michael Bauer and Rhonda Nay, "Family and Staff Partnerships in Long-Term Care: A Review of the Literature," *Journal of Gerontological Nursing* 29, no. 10 (2003): 49.
9. Susan P. Frampton, Laura Gilpin, and Patrick A. Charmel, *Putting Patients First: Designing and Practicing Patient-Centered Care* (San Francisco: Jossey-Bass, 2003), 54.
10. Leslie A. Grant, "Organizational Predictors of Family Satisfaction in Nursing Facilities," *Seniors Housing and Care Journal* 12, no. 1 (2004): 3.
11. Karl Pillemer, J. Jill Suitor, Charles R. Henderson, Jr., Rhoda Meador, Leslie Schultz, Julie Robison, and Carol Hegeman, "A Cooperative Communication Intervention for Nursing Home Staff and Family Members of Residents," *The Gerontologist* 43, special issue 2I (2003): 96–106.
12. Carolyn L. Lindgren and Anne Marie Murphy, "Nurses' and Family Members' Perceptions of Nursing Home Residents' Needs," *Journal of Gerontological Nursing* 28, no. 8 (2002): 52.

CHAPTER 10

1. See Beth Baker, "Aging Well," *Washington Post*, Health section, February 24, 2004.
2. Alzheimer's Association, *www.alz.org*.

3.   Kitwood, *Dementia Reconsidered*, 133.

4.   Ibid., 86.

5.   Tatyana Gurvich and Janet A. Cunningham, "Appropriate Use of Psychotropic Drugs in Nursing Homes," *American Family Physician* 61, no. 5 (2000): 1437–46.

6.   Lon S. Schneider, Pierre N. Tariot, Karen S. Dagerman, et al, "Effectiveness of Atypical Antipsychotic Drugs in Patients with Alzheimer's Disease, *New England Journal of Medicine* 355, no 15 (2006): 1525.

7.   "Jason Karlawish, "Alzheimer's Disease – Clinical Trials and the Logic of Clinical Purpose, " *New England Journal of Medicine* 355, no. 15 (2006): 1604.

8.   Jane Fossey, Clive Ballard, Edmund Juszczak, Ian James, Nicola Alder, Robin Jacoby, and Robert Howard, "Effect of Enhanced Psychosocial Care on Antipsychotic Use in Nursing Home Residents with Severe Dementia: Cluster Randomised Trial," *British Medical Journal* 332 (2006): 756–61.

9.   Margaret P. Calkins and Paul K. Chafetz, "Structuring Environments for Patients with Dementia," in *The Dementias: Diagnosis and Management*, vol. 2 (Washington D.C.: American Psychiatric Press, 1996), 299–300.

10. John Zeisel, Nina M. Silverstein, Joan Hyde, Sue Levkoff, M. Powell Lawton, and William Holmes, "Environmental Correlates to Behavioral Health Outcomes in Alzheimer's Special Care Units," *The Gerontologist* 43, no 5 (2003): 709.

11. Joanne Koenig Coste, *Learning to Speak Alzheimer's: A Groundbreaking Approach for Everyone Dealing with the Disease* (Boston: Houghton Mifflin, 2003), 9.

12. Rebecca McGarry Logue, "Maintaining Family Connectedness in Long-Term Care: An Advanced Practice Approach to Family-Centered Nursing Homes," *Journal of Gerontological Nursing* 29, no. 6 (2003): 28–29.

CHAPTER 11

The first epigraph is from Nursing Home Community Coalition of New York State, "What Makes for a Good Working Condition for Nursing Home Staff: What Do Direct Care Workers Have to Say?" June 2003, *www.ltccc.org/documents/Working ConditionsBooklet_000.pdf.*

1.   The quote is from Debra Parker-Oliver, "Hospice Experience and Perceptions in Nursing Homes," *Journal of Palliative Medicine* 5, no. 5 (2002): 713. For U.S. statistics and deaths in hospitals, Sandra H. Johnson, "Making Room for Dying: End of Life Care in Nursing Homes," *Hastings Center Report*, Special Report 35, *Improving End of Life Care: Why Has It Been So Difficult?* (November–December 2005), no. 6: S37. For the Brown University study, see Debra L. DeSilva, Johanne E. Dillon, and Joan M. Teno, "The Quality of Care in the Last Month of Life among Rhode Island Nursing Home Residents," *Medicine and Health/Rhode Island* 84, no. 6 (2001): 195.

2.   Johnson, "Making Room for Dying," S39.

3.   Barbara M. Raudonis, Ferne C. N. Kyba, and Terri A. Kinsey, "Long-Term Care Nurses' Knowledge of End-of-Life Care," *Geriatric Nursing* 23, no. 6 (2002): 296.

4. Johnson, "Making Room for Dying," S37.
5. Ira Byock, *Dying Well: Peace and Possibilities at the End of Life* (New York: Riverhead Books, 1997), 27.
6. Diane Stillman, Neville Strumpf, Elizabeth Capezuti, and Howard Tuch, "Staff Perceptions Concerning Barriers and Facilitators to End-of-Life Care in the Nursing Home," *Geriatric Nursing* 26, no. 4 (2005): 259.
7. Kathleen M. Davidson, "Evidence-Based Protocol: Family Bereavement Support before and after the Death of a Nursing Home Resident," ed. Jane Hsiao-Chen Tang and Marita G. Titler, *Journal of Gerontological Nursing* 29, no. 1 (2003): 10–18.
8. Sheryl Zimmerman, P. D. Sloane, L. Hanson, C. M. Mitchell, and A. Shy, "Staff Perceptions of End-of-Life Care in Long-Term Care," *Journal of the American Medical Directors Association* 4 (2003): 23–26.
9. Raudonis, Kyba, and Kinsey, "Long-Term Care Nurses' Knowledge," 299.

PART III

The epigraph quoting Bill Keane is from Bill Keane, "The Death of Culture Change?" *Nursing Homes*, November 2005, at *www.nursinghomesmagazine.com*.

CHAPTER 12

1. Kane, "Long-Term Care and a Good Quality of Life," 297.
2. Marilyn Rantz, "Does Good Quality Care in Nursing Homes Cost More or Less than Poor Quality Care?" *Nursing Outlook* 51, no. 2 (2003): 93–94.
3. Bernadette Wright, "Nursing Home Liability Insurance: An Overview," AARP Public Policy Institute, July 2003, *www.aarp.org/research/longtermcare/nursinghomes/*.
4. California Advocates for Nursing Home Reform, "Much Ado about Nothing: Debunking the Myth of Frequent and Frivolous Elder Abuse Lawsuits against California's Nursing Homes," November 2003, 6, *www.canhr.org/pdfs/CANHR_Litigation_Report.pdf*.
5. Philip J, Moore, Nancy E. Adler, and Patricia A. Robertson, "Medical Malpractice: The Effect of Doctor-Patient Relations on Medical Patient Perceptions and Malpractice Intentions," *Western Journal of Medicine* 173 (2000): 244–50.
6. Written communication from Wesley Village, June 30, 2006.
7. Charlene K. Boyd, "The Providence Mount St. Vincent Experience," in *Culture Change in Long-Term Care*, 245–68.
8. Mary Thoesen Coleman, Stephen Looney, James O'Brien, Craig Ziegler, Cynthia A. Pastorino, and Carolyn Turner, "The Eden Alternative: Findings After 1 Year of Implementation," *Journal of Gerontology* 57A, no. 7 (2002): M422.
9. Marian Deutschman, "Redefining Quality and Excellence in the Nursing Home Culture," *Journal of Gerontological Nursing* 27, no. 8 (2001): 29.
10. See *www.achca.org*.

Index

National Alliance for Caregiving, 153
National Citizens' Coalition for Nursing
    Home Reform (NCCNHR), ix, 15, 16,
    22, 23, 116, 156, 192, 193, 205
National Commission on Quality Long-Term
    Care, 203
naturally-occurring retirement communities
    (NORCs), 206
nature, health benefits of, 1, 91, 218
Neel, Armon B., Jr., 19
neglect of nursing home residents, 2, 19, 156,
    164, 203, 212; "The Faces of Neglect:
    Behind the Closed Doors of Nursing
    Homes," 192. *See also* abuse of nursing
    home residents
*Nobody's Home: Candid Reflections of a
    Nursing Home Aide* (Gass), 31, 61, 161,
    175
nonprofit nursing homes, 3, 10, 12, 16, 69, 98,
    186, 196, 201, 202
Norko, Julie, 120
"normalcy" in nursing home life, 16, 45, 90,
    110, 111, 121, 122, 190
Norton, LaVrene, 3, 26–27, 29, 31–32, 60,
    122, 202
Novartis Pharmaceuticals, 68
Novotny, Willie, 43–44
nurses, registered, 18, 19, 71; as supervisors,
    58, 64, 68, 69, 71, 73–75; end-of-life
    care, 175, 177, 180; holistic care, 148; in
    transformational homes, 59, 76, 78–79,
    80–81, 87, 111, 118, 202; resistant to
    change, 59, 68, 73, 117–18. *See also* staff
    turnover
nurse's station, doing away with, 36, 43, 44,
    86–87, 99, 101, 195
"Nursing Home," poem (Morrison), 150
Nursing Home Community Coalition of New
    York State, 67–68, 71
*Nursing Home Design: Consequences of the
    Medical Model* (Schwarz), 4, 100
nursing home history, 10–13; reform
    movement, 13–17
Nursing Home in American Society, The
    (Johnson and Grant), 32. *See also*
    Johnson, Colleen; Grant, Leslie
Nursing Homes magazine, 201
Nursing Home Reform Law, 15–17, 29, 45,
    55, 67, 156, 192, 211–13

nursing home statistics, deaths in, 174;
    number of, 7, 17; projected residents,
    8, 18; residents without family, 113;
    workforce, 8. *See also* costs

Oatfield Estates (Portland, Oregon), 101–2,
    147, 159, 167–68, 202
obstacles to change, 185–99
Olmstead decision, 17
ombudsmen, long-term care, 13, 156, 157,
    211, 213; complaint data, 18–19, 63;
    involvement in culture change, 20, 159,
    160, 203
Omnibus Budget Reconciliation Act of 1987
    (OBRA). *See* Nursing Home Reform
    Law

Pace, Doug, 202
Paraprofessional Healthcare Institute, 73
Parmelee, Patricia A., 20, 28, 36
Partners in Caregiving, 157
Peck, Richard, 201
person- or resident-centered care, 14, 16, 27,
    49, 54, 70, 74, 99, 165–66, 197, 201. *See
    also* resident-directed care; choice
personal growth, resident and employee, 4,
    14, 36, 72, 119, 139, 183, 198, 199, 214,
    215, 216
Petitjean, Noel, 58–59
pets, 1, 22, 33, 91, 93, 94, 95, 96, 110, 133,
    143, 147–48, 150, 195, 218
Pioneer Network, 3, 23, 98, 144, 151, 185,
    198, 202, 206, 207; values and principles,
    214
Pipher, Mary, 200
Planetree, 14, 46, 91, 92, 119, 149, 156, 195,
    202, 216–18. *See also* Wesley Village
Platts-Comeau, Barbara, 55–56, 119
Pleasant View (Concord, N.H.), 55–56, 59,
    118–19, 136–37, 142, 144–45, 146, 147,
    189
Power, Al, 164, 165, 176, 186, 189
pressure sores (bedsores), 17, 32, 35, 50, 52,
    68, 76, 78, 165, 187, 195, 196
privacy, lack of, 9, 18, 29–30, 32, 46, 48, 61,
    87, 117; private rooms, 80, 89, 95, 100,
    146, 159; right to or longing for, 16, 28,
    29, 100, 212, 216
Providence Mount St. Vincent, "the Mount,"

Stevenson, Karen, 11–12
Stevenson, David, 194
Stinson, Jim, 149, 180–81
Stitelman, Martha, 35, 138, 150
St. John's Home (Rochester, N.Y.), 164, 165, 169, 176, 186, 189
Stone, Robyn, 71, 77, 186
stress, 115–16, 131, 148; aides experiencing, 57, 68, 80, 117; consequence of nursing home life, 32, 47–48, 217; family caregivers, 153, 154
Strumpf, Neville, 16

Taft, Lois, 139
technology, 16, 87, 101–102, 203, 206
temporary employees. *See* agency staff
Tender Loving Greed (Mendelson), 15
Teresian House (Albany, N.Y.), 91, 127, 134, 143
That Time of Year: A Chronicle of Life in a Nursing Home. See Joyce Horner
Thieriot, Angelica, 14
Thomas, Barbara, 131, 171, 206
Thomas, Jude, 1, 79, 91
Thomas, W.I., 114
Thomas, William (Bill), ix, 1, 22, 30, 34, 71, 79–80, 88, 90–92, 114, 117, 122, 147, 185–86, 201, 207; "three plagues," 30, 104, 114, 215
Tilly, Jane, 165–66
Tiniacos, Hipp, 94, 112, 113, 173, 174, 177, 180
Tipping Point, The (Gladwell), 200
Tobin, Sheldon S. 116, 185
Tough Guys, 54
Touhy, Theris A., 148
transformational homes.
    See culture change
Turner, Dyke, 92, 132

Ulrich, Roger, 91, 92
universal design, 206. *See also* technology

Unloving Care: The Nursing Home Tragedy. See Bruce Vladeck
Untie the Elderly Campaign. *See* Kendal
U.S. Bureau of Labor Statistics, 63, 65
U.S. Government Accountability Office, 9
veterans and Veterans Administration homes, 12, 34, 47, 76, 101, 138, 150–51, 202

Village, The (Indianola, Iowa), 29, 30, 32, 41, 85–87, 109
Vladeck, Bruce, 9, 12, 15, 17
Voices for Quality Care, 203
volunteers in nursing homes, 24, 78, 92, 93, 97, 110, 117, 119–20, 124, 126–27, 133, 139, 149, 155, 176, 177, 204, 216; residents who volunteer, 113, 144–46, 218

Waldron, Stephanie, 162
Walsh, Joyce, 120
Webb, Juanita, 131, 134
Weldon, Fay, 5
Wellspring, 75, 78
Wesley Village, 105, 119–20, 139, 149, 158, 180–81, 195, 198, 202
West, Joan C., 142
Westphal, Mary Jo, 78
What Are Old People For? (Thomas), 79, 122
Whitley, Joan, 133
Why Zebras Don't Get Ulcers (Sapolsky), 48
Wright, Bernadette, 193
Why Survive? Being Old in America (Butler), 15
Williams, Carter Catlett, 16, 22, 23, 101, 151, 200
Wilson, Marsha, 58, 76, 180

Zimmerman, Sheryl, 128, 177, 196
Zweibel, Nancy, 140, 204